DETOX

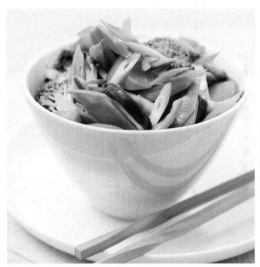
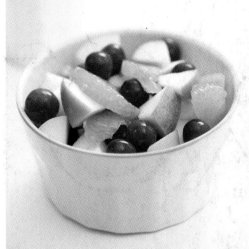
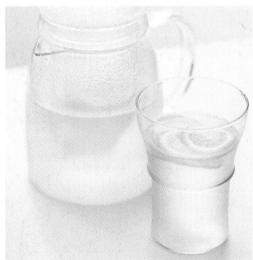
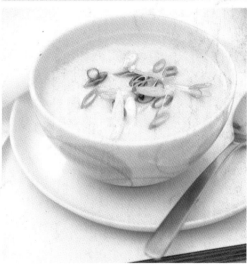

THE AUSTRALIAN Women's Weekly

Looking healthy and feeling good about myself are important to me... that's why every now and then I need a bit of a tune-up. Detoxing is not a flash in the pan like so many other diets, but a healthy, sensible way to help rid yourself of many of the harmful things you take into your body simply by living in the world today. And guess what? The food in this book is so delicious, it may well become food you want to eat all the time.

Pamela Clark

Food Director

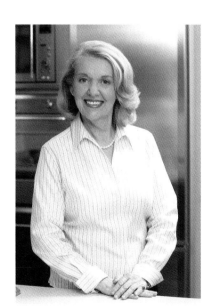

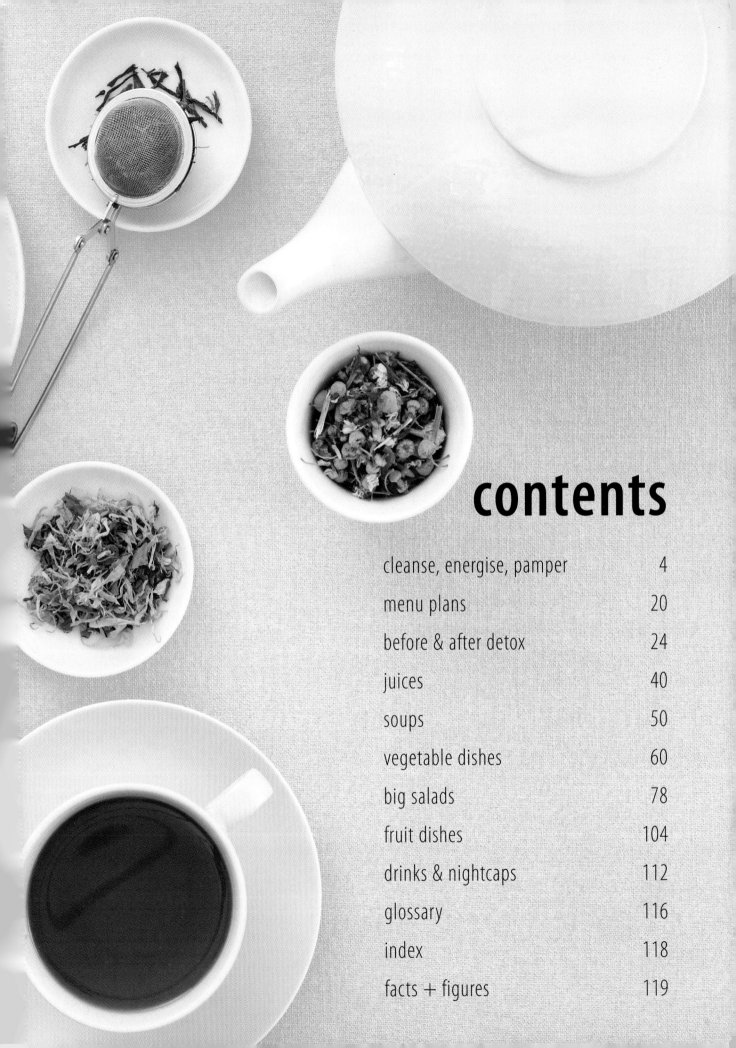

contents

cleanse, energise, pamper	4
menu plans	20
before & after detox	24
juices	40
soups	50
vegetable dishes	60
big salads	78
fruit dishes	104
drinks & nightcaps	112
glossary	116
index	118
facts + figures	119

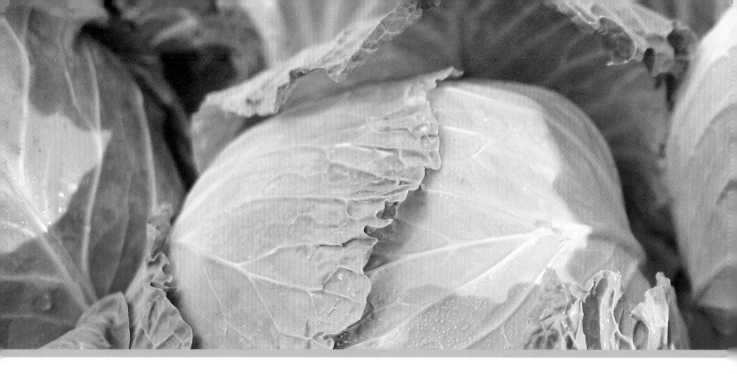

cleanse, energise, pamper

WHY YOU NEED TO DETOX

We all want to enjoy good health, unlimited energy, restful sleep and a sense of serenity. But increasingly the world around us presents us with some real challenges in realising these goals.

We may find ourselves relying on convenience food to meet our nutritional needs because we're working longer hours. Is it any wonder, then, that our freezers tend to be stocked with frozen dinners or other convenience-oriented food, or that we find ourselves dialling takeaway more often than is healthy? And, even if we try to improve our diet, buying natural produce and ingredients isn't as easy as it once was. Many supermarket shelves are stocked with foods grown or raised with the use of pesticides and antibiotics, that contain artificial additives or preservatives, or have had much of the goodness processed out of them.

It's been estimated that, on average, we eat or drink about 3.75 litres of pesticides, take in five kilograms of chemical food additives and breathe in two grams of solid pollution every year.

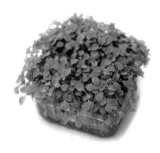

At the same time, the water that comes out of our taps contains chemical contaminants, and the air we breathe is polluted with toxins from industry, transportation and even the cleaning products we use around our homes.

These all have toxic effects – the Environmental Protection Agency in the United States considers that 60 per cent of all herbicides, 90 per cent of all fungicides and 30 per cent of all insecticides are potentially carcinogenic (cancer-causing).

Besides external sources, toxins in our body can result from viral or bacterial infections, or from the by-products of the metabolism of certain bacteria and yeasts that inhabit our bowel.

As if this isn't enough for our bodies to deal with, nearly all of us find ourselves locked into a hyperactive state, with very little time to spend in a healing state, where we can let go of stress. We also relegate stress-beating exercise to the bottom of our to-do list.

To fight this combination of challenges, many of us turn to medical or recreational drugs to combat ills or help us unwind. But, ironically, these further pollute our bodies, causing more toxins and stress.

Unfortunately, the payoff for our 21st-century lifestyle is excess weight, allergies, headaches, fatigue, rashes, colds, coughs and a host of other ailments.

Yet there is some good news. Our body is an incredible feat of biomechanical engineering. All we need do is give it the tools – and that includes a "detox" – to repair the damage wreaked by an overload of toxins, and it will put us back onto the path to wellbeing.

What we need is a program that will cleanse and energise our body and mind, and help us build a healthy lifestyle – and that includes some self-pampering.

The benefits are many: increased energy, glowing skin, healthier hair and nails, less anxiety, better concentration, better metabolism and bowel patterns and, in the long-term, a slowing down of the ageing process and a lower risk of both minor illnesses and chronic disease.

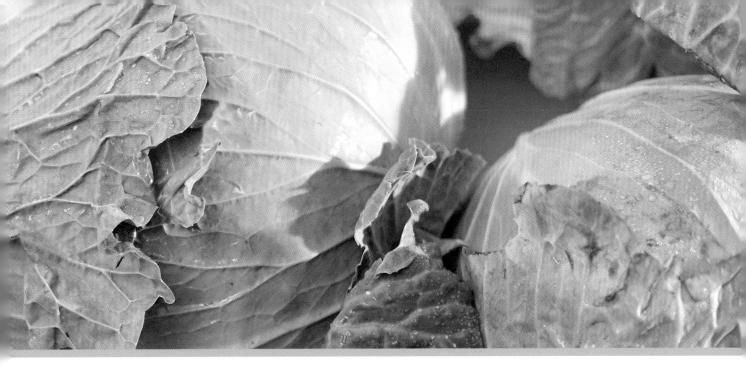

HOW YOU KNOW YOU NEED TO DETOX

If you are in tune with your body, you will often feel when it's not running smoothly.

But even if you've lost touch with your personal rhythms, your body will send you plenty of signals that it needs a detox tune-up. (See the "symptoms" checklist, right.)

WHEN TO DETOX – AND WHEN NOT TO

Detoxing can be challenging, so you need to choose a time that works for you. The start of spring, summer or autumn are best, because you don't need as much food to refuel your body as you do in winter, and detox foods tend to be light. Ideally, you should also choose a time when you're not under a lot of pressure or, better still, when you have a few days off – it's important that you take it easy.

Directly after a bout of the flu or food poisoning is a bad time to detox. So, wait until you've had sufficient time to recover.

You may also want to delay starting a detox program if you are feeling emotionally vulnerable – such as if you've just ended a relationship or moved house.

While many people choose the longer detox programs – seven days or two weeks – you should be aware that you may face some hurdles in maintaining your busy schedule. For example, you may develop a detox headache and find it difficult to concentrate. We recommend that you don't take painkillers because they add to your toxic load.

Be aware that withdrawal headaches from caffeine, which is on the "foods to avoid" list (page 9), can be particularly vicious on the second day. You'll need to make sure you drink plenty of water and that, if you want

DO YOU NEED TO DETOX?

How many of these symptoms apply to you?
- · You're always tired and don't sleep well
- · You suffer from breakouts or dull skin
- · You are constipated or suffer from irritable bowel syndrome
- · Your eyes are puffy and accentuated with dark circles
- · You often feel nauseous or suffer from indigestion
- · You have aches and pains in your joints or muscles
- · You are prone to sinus problems or allergies
- · You just can't get rid of cellulite
- · You have skin that is dry and itchy
- · Your hair is dull or greasy
- · You suffer from headaches
- · You suffer from night sweats
- · You have bad breath
- · You suffer from flatulence
- · You have recurrent itchy or inflamed eyes
- · Bloating and water retention are a problem for you
- · You often lose your train of thought
- · Your moods are up and down
- · You feel anxious or depressed
- · You suffer from skin rashes or eczema
- · You're so stressed you want to scream

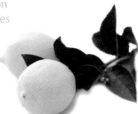

to, you can lie down until the effects of the headache subsides.

If you feel light-headed on a detox program never drive a car or operate machinery. Rest is the best remedy.

Also, avoid very hot baths and showers, as these not only reduce your energy, but may increase your blood pressure.

We recommend you stop the detox program immediately if you feel sick, light-headed or dizzy, or if you have a constant headache or muscle pain that you would rate as severe. Don't feel discouraged. You can always embark on the program again when you feel more able.

NOTE: Detoxing is not suitable for pregnant women or people with diabetes, kidney disease, or eating disorders. Those with any medical condition that requires regular supervision by their doctor or prescribed medication should also seek their GP's advice before embarking on any program that involves a change of eating or exercise habits.

CLEANING UP

Ever wondered how the body disposes of the toxic waste accumulated in your system? Toxins are cleansed from the body in a variety of ways, but mainly through:

· your liver, for final elimination through your lungs, kidneys and intestines
· your lungs, which exhale poisonous carbon dioxide and other waste products
· your kidneys, which eliminate water-soluble toxins
· your intestines, which eliminate both water and fat-soluble toxins and wastes
· your skin, through perspiration
· your hair and nails, which eliminate some toxins, including heavy metals

PREPARING TO DETOX

You'll notice that we've included some "day before" advice in the one-week detox menu, and some "two-days before" guidelines for the two-week program. That's because you need to ease into the program to reduce sudden withdrawal symptoms.

If you drink six cups of coffee a day and go straight onto water or herbal tea, we're pretty sure you're going to have a headache that will put you off ever undertaking a detox program again. A week before you're due to start detoxing, cut your caffeine intake by a cup a day. If you drink alcohol or eat a lot of sugar, drink or eat them less and less as the days to your detox approach.

Setting up your environment to detox is also very important. Throw out any foods that are full of sugar, caffeine, white flour or saturated and trans fats (a "bad" fat that raises cholesterol levels; usually found in cakes, biscuits and table margarines).

Ask yourself if that king-sized chocolate bar will survive your detox or whether you'll be tempted by that cup of coffee. Remember, after you've finished your detox, you'll be making healthier food choices. You'll need to replace unhealthy foods with healthy ones – lots of fruit and vegetables, filtered water, herbal teas and pulses and grains. See our menus (pages 20-23) and make a shopping list. Wherever possible, buy organic so your body won't have to deal with the chemicals used on commercial fruits and vegetables.

You'll also need some essential kitchen tools: a steamer and juice extractor (borrow one if you haven't got one), for example, so you can get the benefits of freshly squeezed oranges, lemons, pineapples and more.

HERO DETOX FOODS

Apples Contain vitamin E, which improves endurance and stamina of muscles and nerves, and protects the respiratory system from toxins. Also a good source of vitamins A and C, biotin, folic acid and quercetin, an antioxidant that helps lower fat and cholesterol.

Beetroot Reputed to be one of the best liver-cleansing vegetables, it also helps nourish the nervous system and brain with manganese, magnesium and folate.

Broccoli Is high in folate and vitamins A and C, as well as calcium and phosphorous, which help build and maintain strong bones. It also stimulates the liver.

Cabbage High in vitamin C and calcium. An excellent source of chlorine and sulphur, which expel waste and cleans the blood.

Carrots Packed with nutrients including vitamins A and C; believed to cleanse, nourish and stimulate the body, particularly the liver, kidneys and digestive system.

Celery A recognised diuretic and laxative, and the richest vegetable source of sodium with more than 120mg per 100 grams.

Cherries Food for the blood with iron, copper and manganese, plus vitamins A and C. They help remove toxins from the kidneys, liver and digestive system. Cherries also contain a phytochemical called ellagic acid, which could help protect against cancer.

Chickpeas A good source of fibre and calcium for healthy bones, phosphorous for healthy kidneys and nerves, and potassium, which nourishes muscles.

Cucumber Contains high levels of vitamin E, essential for healthy heart muscles, and iodine for healthy hair, nails, skin, teeth and thyroid function. Helps prevent water retention.

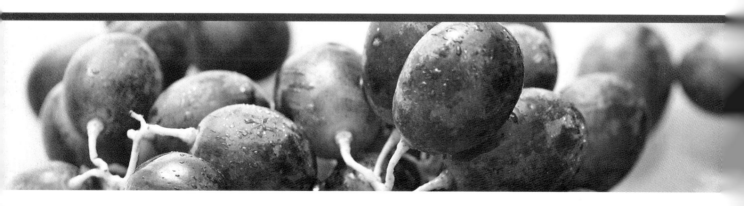

Fennel A diuretic that can also help settle the stomach.

Garlic A powerhouse of sulphur, a natural penicillin that helps keep the body alkaline. Garlic oil contains a substance that helps clear the respiratory and lymphatic system.

Ginger Cleans, stimulates and rejuvenates the digestive system.

Grapes Contain ellagic acid that may have anti-carcinogenic effects. Also contains high levels of manganese, the "memory mineral", which nourishes the nervous system, helps maintain sex hormone production and assists in the formation of healthy red blood cells. A good source of silicon, which helps circulation, prevents nervous exhaustion and is essential for healthy skin, hair and teeth.

Lemons An excellent source of phosphorous, required for the repair and healthy functioning of the nervous system. Also a good source of sodium, which assists in the proper elimination of waste and cleansing of the lymphatic system, and helps stimulate the liver and gallbladder. Freshly squeezed lemon juice in warm water (ratio 25/75) first thing in the morning is a great way to pep up your liver.

Melons High in sodium to help cleanse the kidneys. Also contain a host of other minerals including calcium, phosphorus, potassium, iron and zinc, as well as vitamins A and C.

Onions A good source of silicon, which can promote better blood circulation and prevent nervous and mental fatigue. Also contain potent antiviral and antibacterial nutrients.

Oranges Loaded with vitamin C, with an average of 30-50mg/100g of freshly squeezed juice. Also contain calcium and phosphorous, which, when combined, help protect the body from infections and viruses.

Papaya One of the richest sources of the enzyme papain, which is essential to protein digestion. Also an excellent source of vitamins A and C.

Parsley Stimulates the kidneys to eliminate toxic waste.

Peaches A good source of vitamin A, important for healthy skin, good eyesight and protection from the effects of stress and environmental toxins. Vitamin A also protects the lungs and respiratory tract from infection. Contain sulphur, which can help expel harmful mucus from the body.

Pears Contain alkaline-healing and cleansing minerals including potassium, sodium, iron calcium, magnesium and manganese. Also contain sodium, which not only benefits the lymphatic system, but is required regularly for proper elimination of carbon dioxide waste from the lungs.

Pineapples Contain bromelain, which has anti-inflammatory properties and helps the body digest protein.

Sea vegetables Alginic acid, found in some seaweeds, binds with heavy metals, such as cadmium, lead, mercury and radium, to eliminate them from the body.

Strawberries Contain ellagic acid that may have anti-carcinogenic effects. Weight for weight, contain 1½ times as much vitamin C as most citrus fruits and are also a good source of iron.

Tomatoes Contain chlorine, an acid mineral that stimulates the liver to filter out waste products. Helps with the production of gastric juices, maintenance of correct fluid levels and the reduction of excess blood fat.

Watercress Reputed to cleanse the blood and improve the condition of the skin.

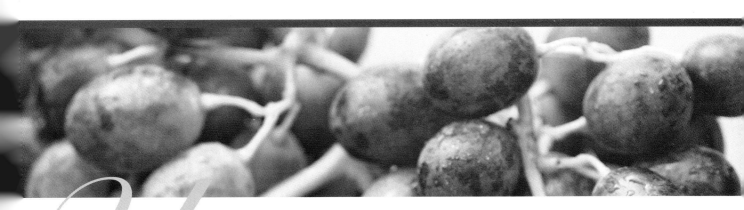

Using beautiful plates, glasses and cutlery during a detox can also increase your sense of pampering yourself.

If it's fresh, organic and a fruit or vegetable, it's an excellent detox food.

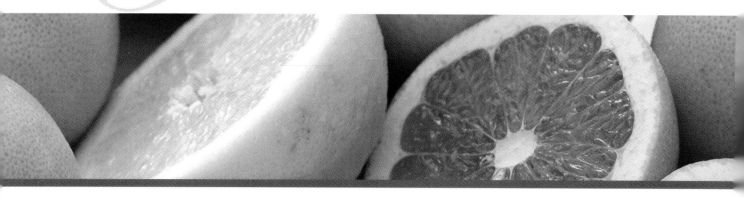

OTHER EXCELLENT DETOX FOODS

Apricots An excellent source of vitamin A, and a good source of vitamin C and fibre.

Avocados Supply all the essential daily B-group vitamins as well as magnesium, calcium, phosphorous and potassium. Are a great source of "good" fats, which help lower cholesterol and glutathione, an antioxidant that combines with fat-soluble toxins to make them water-soluble.

Bananas Very high in potassium, and a great source of the "memory mineral", manganese, as well as iron and copper for healthy blood, magnesium, calcium and phosphorous, vitamins A and C, and some B-group vitamins.

Barley The wholegrain variety is a good source of B vitamins and also contains a host of minerals that are nourishing and cleansing. It is also high in fibre.

Grapefruit A great source of vitamins C and E, and some of the B-group vitamins.

Lentils Very low in fat and full of iron, zinc, magnesium, vitamin A and B-group vitamins. Also high in fibre.

Lettuce Supplies more than 2000mg/100g of the mineral silicon, which helps promote calcium metabolism and eliminates excess uric acid deposits from the bone structure and bloodstream. Go for the darker green leaves.

Prunes Have high levels of magnesium, which have a natural laxative effect. Good supply of potassium. Help the blood become more alkaline.

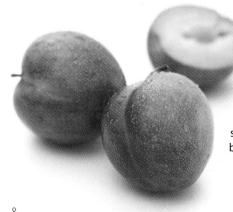

Pumpkin An excellent source of bone-building silicon, as well as vitamin A, which is necessary for good vision, healthy skin and a strong immune system. Pumpkin is also a good source of vitamin C, potassium, iron and is high in fibre.

Spinach Contains chlorine, which regulates correct acid and alkali levels in the blood, as well as silicon, sodium, vitamins A and E, magnesium, manganese, copper and iron.

Sesame seeds An excellent source of protein, calcium, iron and magnesium. Also assist in the formation of blood platelets and, in combination with iron, have blood purifying qualities.

Tofu As well as being low in saturated fat and a vegetarian source of protein, tofu seems to have the ability to bind to heavy metals, so they can be eliminated from the body.

Yogurt Natural yogurt contains good bacteria that can help cleanse the digestive system and keep intestinal flora healthy.

FOODS TO AVOID

Toxins are harmful substances that affect the healthy functioning of our bodies. Most people are aware that their diet needs improving and, by controlling what they eat, they can control some of the toxins that enter their body.

The following should be regarded as "toxins-on-a-plate": chemical preservatives, dyes, flavouring agents, additives, artificial sweeteners and hydrogenated vegetable oils. Make sure you avoid them.

Also avoid processed and refined foods that have had their natural nutrients stripped and destroyed. Wherever possible, a better choice is organic whole foods.

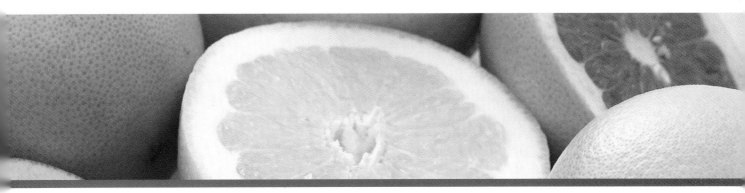

Most people who detox should also cut out meat, wheat and dairy. Naturopaths believe these foods create acid toxins that, in excess, can damage organs and glands, harm joints and arteries, and even inhibit immune responses.

Unfortunately, many dairy foods and meats now contain growth promoters, hormones and antibiotics that put a strain on the whole body. However, one exception is natural live yogurt, which has a soothing and nurturing effect on the digestive system, and can help keep healthy bacteria in the gut. We use sheep- or goats-milk yogurt in our recipes, as these are much easier to digest and can aid digestive disorders and stimulate digestion.

Meat is also hard to digest, and is a major source of saturated fat, the kind that will contribute to blocked arteries and increase the risk of heart disease.

You'll notice we don't include fish in our detox programs, because it can harbour unwanted pollutants. But, even though we want you to stick to a vegetarian diet while cleansing and re-energising your body, you may want to incorporate fish later into your diet, and so we have included fish in the "before & after" section of the menus. In fact, most health experts recommend that you eat three servings of fish a week because of its ability to reduce the risk of heart disease, and auto-immune and joint problems.

Two other things you won't be allowed on a detox are wheat and alcohol.

Wheat is a common allergen and wheat bran can inhibit the absorption of some important nutrients, as well as irritate the intestinal lining.

In large quantities, alcohol can be a toxic substance, and heavy drinking can harm the liver and deplete nutrients such as vitamins A and C and the B-group vitamins, as well as magnesium, zinc and essential fatty acids. It can lead to severe dehydration. Modern methods of producing alcohol also means it often contains chemical pesticides, colorants and other harmful additives.

Bad news for cappuccino addicts: caffeine is also on the "foods to avoid" list, as are sugar and salt. Consuming an excessive amount of caffeine can result in insomnia, headaches and high blood pressure, as well as reducing the body's ability to absorb vitamins and minerals.

Of course, large amounts of refined sugar not only upset the balance of blood sugars in the body, but are full of empty kilojoules.

Salt is necessary to maintain normal hydration of the body's circulation and cellular fluids. However, many people eat too much salt, simply because food manufacturers tend to add salt to everyday foods such as bread, cereals and canned goods. Too much salt overloads the kidneys and can cause fluid retention, which may lead to heart failure, stroke, osteoporosis or kidney problems, including kidney stones.

In our detox recipes, we've used fresh herbs and lemon juice to add zest to food. We're sure you'll also find these healthier alternatives just as flavoursome.

FOODS TO AVOID

- processed & refined foods
- hydrogenated vegetable oils
- wheat
- alcohol
- caffeine
- dairy
- fish
- salt
- sugar
- meat

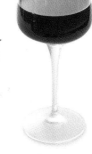

Rather than use salt, a better way to flavour foods and give it zest, is to add fresh herbs and lemon juice.

Drink like a fish during your detox... but make it nothing but juice, water and herbal tea.

GETTING THE BALANCE RIGHT

The acid/alkaline level of the body (also known as the "Ph" level) is important for healthy cells and tissues. For the body to function properly, it needs to keep its acid/alkaline balance within normal levels. If the body is too acid or too alkaline, cells can be damaged and tissues won't function effectively, thereby affecting your health.

Foods can affect the Ph level of the body (which is normally slightly alkaline), and diet appears to be one of the causes of an unbalanced Ph level. Some foods break down into acid-forming substances, while others break down into alkaline-forming substances. The diet of many people in Western countries consists of acid-forming food (saturated fats, sugar, meat, processed foods and refined products), therefore the body has a more acid Ph level than is healthy.

Your diet should be made up of 70 per cent alkali-forming foods and 30 per cent acid-forming foods. Alkaline-forming foods consist of most fresh fruits, including citrus, melons, pineapple, mango, kiwifruit and papaya, and vegetables, including asparagus, celery, spinach, carrot, onion, broccoli and potatoes (with the skin on). Acid-forming foods include meats, fish, poultry, eggs, cheese, bread, rice, oats, most cereals, lentils, sugar, walnuts and hazelnuts.

Naturopaths believe that keeping your body in an alkaline state will improve your mood, energy levels, sleep quality, and reduce aches and pains, headaches and, in the long-term, your risk of chronic disease.

Exercise also can affect the acid/alkaline balance of your body by making the blood more acidic. Deep breathing, on the other hand, makes the blood more alkaline.

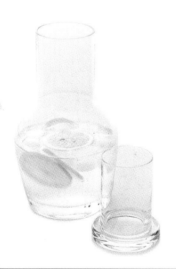

H2O

Drink like a fish during your detox, but make it nothing but juice, water and herbal tea. Sixty per cent of your body is made up of fluid, which is absolutely essential for the healthy functioning of your entire system.

Fluids promote chemical reactions, lubricate joints, transport nutrients and are important for kidney and immune function, healthy skin, and even the prevention of pain.

You need to drink 1-1.5 litres of pure water a day. You can add a squeeze of lemon juice to it if you wish. And you'll find plenty of delicious juices included in the detox plans.

But don't just use water on the inside to purify your body. The section on External Detoxing (page 11) explains how to cleanse your body with H2O on the outside.

EXERCISE AND DETOX

True or false. If you swim, go for a run or have a workout at the gym, you will detox faster. *False.* In fact, indulging in this sort of strenuous exercise while you're on a detox program could land you in hospital. A detox is not the time to run a marathon.

No matter what detox program you choose to undertake, it's important you get plenty of rest. If you're on the one-day detox program, the most strenuous thing you should do is have a massage. If you choose the weekend detox, a bit of gentle walking is the only exercise recommended. For the one- and two-week detox programs, two gentle walks a week are all you need to help eliminate toxins such as urea and lactic acid.

An alternative to walking is five or 10 minutes of gentle exercise, such as yoga, tai chi and chi gong. These exercises gently pump lymph, an alkaline fluid that removes acid waste from the blood and tissues, around the body. Gentle exercise also helps dissolve and eliminate crystalline acid deposits in the joints.

Remember, there is no compulsion to exercise. In fact, on the stricter fasts, experts recommend against it. If you feel you need extra sleep, or you simply want to lie down, it is important you follow your body's cues. Lounge around at home, if possible, assign household tasks to someone else, and try to avoid attending social functions. The whole idea is to let your body restore and regenerate.

PAMPER YOURSELF

While you're cleansing your inside with detoxing foods and juices, it's the ideal time to cleanse and pamper your outside, too.

DRY BODY BRUSHING AND AN EPSOM SALTS BATH

Dry body brushing is a stimulating therapy. It's a great detoxing treatment because it helps rid the skin of dry, dead cells and improves blood and lymph circulation. That means it helps your body dispose of some of the internal toxins being mobilised by your detox program.

You'll need a natural bristle brush or a hemp mitt. Undress then, on dry skin, use long, upward sweeping movements, starting at your feet and working up your legs and across your hips and bottom (the strokes should be towards your heart). From there, run the brush in a clockwise motion over your stomach then gently rub over your decolletage area and down your arms to your fingers.

Don't brush your breasts, face or throat, and be careful not to rub your skin too hard. Rough scrubbing can break tiny capillaries, not to mention leave you red and raw.

After you've finished dry brushing you can have shower, or you may want to run a warm bath and put in one to two cups of Epsom salts – available from chemists or supermarkets. These contain magnesium, a mineral required for nearly all the body's cellular activity, and is especially important to healthy muscle function.

An Epsom salts bath will stimulate lymph drainage and draw toxins out through the pores on the skin. For maximum detoxing benefits, soak about 20 minutes. Afterwards, it is recommended that you drink plenty of water and relax for an hour, as an Epsom salts bath can be quite draining.

For best results, take an Epsom salts bath every three days during a detox program. However, you shouldn't have one if you suffer from a skin condition, or have any cuts.

AROMATHERAPY

There are few more luxurious ways to help you detox, as well as stimulate your senses, revive your soul and heal your mind and body, than aromatherapy.

While many people might think of aromatherapy simply as a form of treatment that involves nice-smelling oils, it is much more than that. The plant-extracted essential oils really do have therapeutic effects. They also can be dangerous if used incorrectly or in the wrong amounts, so always follow the instructions.

SOME ESSENTIAL OILS AND THEIR USES

Bergamot	relieves stress, depression and fatigue
Cedarwood	comforting, helps calm the nerves
Chamomile	calms the nerves
Clary sage	helps relieve stress, tension and mild anxiety
Eucalyptus	can help relieve cold and flu symptoms
Fennel	detoxifying, good for digestive problems, tiredness
Frankincense	helps bring comfort
Geranium	helps calm the nerves, relieves anxiety and tension
Grapefruit	detoxifying, uplifting
Ginger	warming and stimulating
Juniper	calming and detoxifying
Lavender	helps relieve insomnia, nervous tension and headache
Lemon	helps relieve the symptoms of colds
Lime	refreshing and reviving
Mandarin	a diuretic, also has sedative properties
Myrrh	has anti-inflammatory properties
Orange	helps relieve stress and tension
Peppermint	clears the head, good for fatigue
Rosemary	uplifting and focusing
Sandalwood	warming and grounding
Tea tree	cleansing, uplifting and refreshing
Ylang ylang	a sedative, calms the nerves

The easiest ways to use aromatherapy oils are in an oil burner or a bath. Using an oil burner is an ideal accompaniment to any relaxation or meditation that you may perform during your detox. Fill the oil-burner dish with water and light the candle. Add about five drops of essential oil to the water (some oils are not suitable for a burner, so check the label before use), and within minutes the aroma from the heated oil will gradually permeate the room.

An aromatherapy bath can feel like a luxurious treat while acting as a great tonic for the body, and the steam from the bath carries more aroma molecules to your nose than when you burn them.

The best way to use essential oils in the bath is to add them a drop at a time, using no more than six to eight drops in a full bath. Don't add more if you can't smell them after a while; they're still working. Also, don't have the water too hot or you may feel light-headed. For the same reason, saunas and steam rooms are not recommended during a detox, although they can be helpful later to keep the body healthy by helping to eliminate toxins.

As you rest in the bath your muscles relax and release lactic acid; your pores open and release toxins in the form of sweat; and your digestive system is stimulated by the heat of the bath. Your open pores allow the essential oil to penetrate your skin more readily. Try one of the essential oil blends (page 13), for a relaxing detox bath.

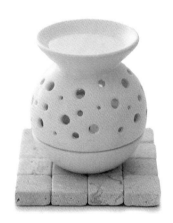

NOTE: All essential oils must be used with caution. Some oils should be avoided by people with certain medical conditions or skin sensitivities, and by those who are pregnant. If you are unsure whether you can use essential oils, it is important to first talk to a qualified naturopathic practitioner or GP. Never take essential oils internally.

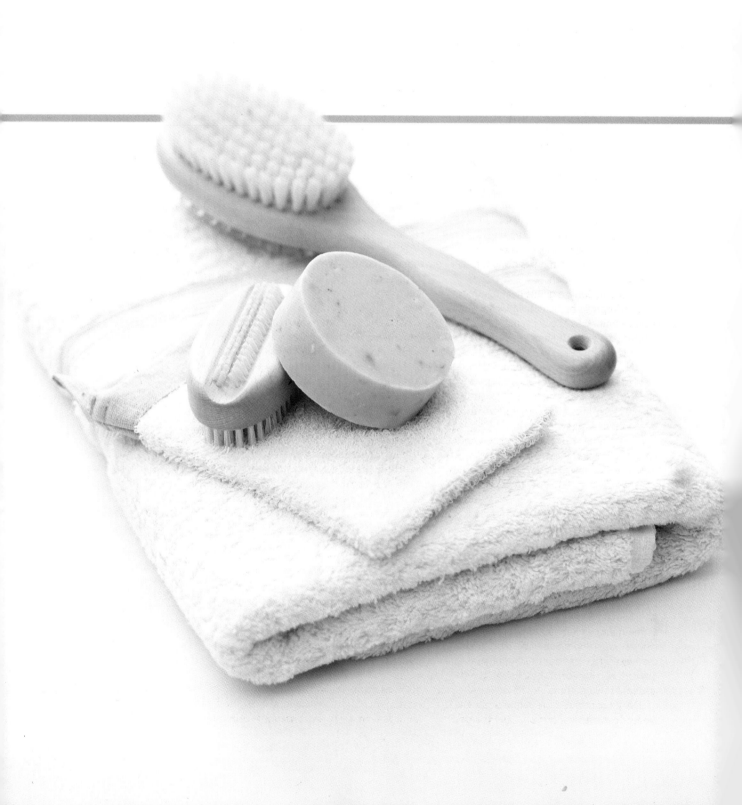

OTHER HYDROTHERAPY TREATMENTS

There are a number of ways to benefit from the power of water other than soaking in it.

Yes, hydrotherapy does include such treatments as an aromatherapy bath, but it can also be more specifically used as a hot and/or cold sitz bath, a hot and/or cold foot bath or a fomentation (the applation of warm liquid to the skin).

The idea is that the body doesn't respond to the water itself, but to the variations in the water temperature – heat dilates the vessels, increases the blood flow and relaxes the nerves and tissues while cold constricts the vessels, reduces the blood flow and stimulates the nerves and tissues.

While a sitz bath requires two tubs, and is too difficult to do at home (although you may want to take the treatment at a salon), a hot and cold foot bath is easy to perform.

You'll need one bucket or bowl of hot water (40°C) and another filled with cold tap water. Place your feet in the hot water first. Wiggle your toes and gently twist your ankles for three minutes while your feet are in the water. Then put your feet into the cold water for one minute. Repeat twice, finishing with the cold water. Then dry your feet briskly. This treatment is good for stimulating circulation.

A fomentation is a gentle heat treatment used to improve blood circulation and waste elimination. It can decrease pain, increase mobility and reduce inflammation of joints or muscles. Fomentations can also be used over the region of various body organs, such as the liver, lungs, kidneys, stomach and lower abdominal area, to speed up the removal of waste products from the tissues.

You'll need 10 towels, a hot-water bottle and, ideally, someone to help lay the towels over you if the area is hard to reach.

Begin by filling the hot-water bottle and wrapping it in one towel; put it aside for a moment. Make sure you're positioned comfortably, perhaps on the floor with pillows to support your body.

Now, place eight layers of towels over the area you wish to be treated. Place the towel-wrapped hot-water bottle on top for three minutes. Remove the hot-water bottle and towels, then take a wet towel (soaked in cold water and wrung out so it doesn't drip) and place it on the area you are treating for one minute. Repeat this procedure two more times, finishing with the cold towel.

Do not continue if the pain increases, and never do more than two treatments a day.

PAMPERING DURING DETOX

Stress is a major contributor to a toxic state, but pampering and relaxation techniques can allow our body to release tension and anxiety.

Reflexology, full-body massages and facials can all help relax the nervous system and speed the elimination of stress-induced toxins from the body. And not only that, they feel great, too.

REFLEXOLOGY

Reflexology is said to stimulate our natural healing abilities and balance and energise our body's systems.

Our feet are considered miniature maps of our bodies, and reflexologists believe that poor diet, stress, lack of exercise and illness can cause congestion in the feet, resulting in deposits of crystalline-like lumps around the nerve endings. These lumps are broken down during treatment by deep finger massage of the feet.

To help them navigate the feet – and the body – reflexologists use a chart that shows which areas and points of the feet correspond to other parts of the body, such as the liver or the sinuses. They then look for tender spots, where they apply pressure to break down any crystalline deposits. These are then eliminated from the body through the bloodstream.

Reflexologists believe that this has a flow-on effect in the body – with the deposits eliminated, the body part they correspond to can become more healthy.

To be your own reflexologist, start with a bath, shower or even a foot soak (try adding a disinfecting essential oil such as lime or lemon). Gently dry your feet, making sure you dry between your toes.

Start with the right foot and use your thumb to "walk" in a straight line along the outside edge of the foot. With each movement of the thumb, press down into the foot – not so that you experience pain, but

Mix your own essential oil bath blend to soothe aching muscles, boost the immune and digestive systems and bring a sense of peace and harmony.

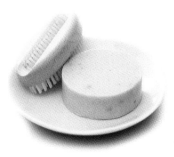

just deep enough to feel a release of tension in the foot. Next, walk the thumb over the ball of the foot in rows until you have covered the area. Then, walk the thumb along the left, middle and right side of each toe.

If you notice any tender spots while you are doing this, don't panic – while they could indicate that you may have some congestion in the corresponding body part, they will become less and less tender if you continue to practice reflexology.

Many people find the arch to be the most tender part of the foot, and this may be particularly true during a detox. Reflexologists claim the arch has many points that correspond to the elimination organs (the lungs, kidneys and bowel). Working on the arch also helps improve circulation, which, in turn, helps the body to remove wastes and toxins more effectively.

> **Learning to breathe properly is an essential part of any self-healing detox program.**

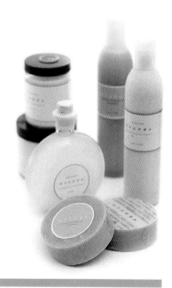

Two drops of cedarwood or eucalyptus essential oil mixed into 4ml of a carrier oil, such as almond oil, and rubbed into your feet while you perform your reflexology treatment will help flush the kidneys and keep your feet fresh.

MASSAGE

For a pleasurable way to knead toxins from the tissues, promote lymph drainage, stimulate glandular secretions and calm the nervous system, try one of the many types of massage. It can relieve tension, help improve the immune system, tone the skin and muscles, and improve the appearance of skin, especially in areas prone to cellulite.

Book a treatment before you start your detox program, but take time to consider which style of massage will suit you best.

You may find a gentle Swedish massage is as much as you feel up to. Or, maybe a deeper therapy, such as remedial massage, is just what you need to get circulation going.

Other options include shiatsu massage, which involves stretching, manipulation and acupressure and can be quite painful (but effective), and kahuna massage, an energetic process that helps connect body and soul.

You can also massage yourself – or at least the parts you can reach. All massage strokes should be towards your heart, pushing the blood around your body in conjunction with the circulation, not against it.

Self-massage isn't quite as relaxing as having someone else do it for you, though. So why not spoil yourself? After all, you are taking time out for you.

BREATHING

If you are what you eat, you're also a product of how you breathe. In fact, learning to breathe properly is an essential part of any self-healing detox program. If the body does not expel sufficient carbon dioxide, toxins build up.

Deep, rhythmic breathing enhances oxygenation of the blood and tissues, and switches the nervous system into the healing mode. By contrast, shallow, overbreathing can put you in a state of anxiety that can lead to ill health.

Try this simple breathing exercise to de-stress and recharge: sit comfortably or lie down. Place your hands gently on your stomach, with your fingertips touching. Close your eyes and take a few normal breaths while you say the word "calm" in your mind.

Now, breathe in through your nose, very slowly, to a count of four. As you inhale, push your belly up and out. Hold your breath for five counts, then gently exhale through your mouth to a count of eight. Repeat this process up to 10 times.

FACIALS

Oh-oh. It's day two of your detox and you look like a teenager again. Don't worry. Breaking out during a cleansing program is normal. And once you've detoxed your body, skin problems should subside. To help your skin clear up, and to add extra relaxation to your detox regime, consider having a facial.

If you decide to visit a salon, make sure you choose somewhere with a relaxing atmosphere. Ask what the treatment includes before you book to make sure it will fit in with your regime. A head or shoulder massage or being left alone with a mask on for 15 minutes are both pluses because they help you relax and give you time for reflection.

If you'd prefer to treat yourself at home, stock up on some of your favourite cleanser, mask and moisturiser products before you start your detox. Or, for a natural treatment, raid the pantry, the kitchen is the ideal place for facial ingredients – you can't go past honey, natural yogurt or oatmeal. Also try your local chemist or health-food store for supplies. These are ideal places to seek out chemical-free beauty products.

A facial sauna is a good way to prepare your face for facial masks. (You should not use facial saunas if you have sensitive skin, are pregnant or suffer from asthma.) Give these facial saunas a try.

Fill a large glass bowl with 1 litre (4 cups) of near boiling water; add ingredients according to your skin type (page 15). Place a towel

over your head and hold it over the bowl from a distance of about 30cm for a period of about 2 minutes. Close your eyes and breathe normally; allow the steam to open your pores. Remove your face from the sauna; pat face with a warm face washer.
Normal skin: add 6 drops mandarin essential oil and 2 tablespoons loose lavender tea to water.
Oily skin: add 6 drops eucalyptus essential oil and 2 tablespoons loose lemon tea to water.
Dry skin: add 6 drops rose essential oil and 2 tablespoons loose chamomile tea to water.

Ideally, perform home treatments when you are alone and have some private time and space – and don't forget to take the phone off the hook. It's all about self-pampering; an indulgence to build into your life, even after you finish your detox program.

POSSIBLE SIDE EFFECTS OF DETOXING

Unfair as it may seem, some people get next to no detoxing symptoms. However, most people will notice some annoying side effects, and these will also vary greatly from person to person.

Detoxing symptoms commonly include headaches, lower back pain, dry mouth, coated tongue, bad breath, skin rashes, nausea, body odour, weakness, fatigue, abdominal gas and rumblings, palpitations, mucous discharges, irritability, boredom, anxiety, emotional upset, joint and muscular aches and pains, cold feet and hands, vivid dreams, sleeplessness and more. As well, existing health problems, such as arthritis, may seem to worsen initially, and the effects of old injuries may also become evident.

The first three or four days is the most common time for reactions and withdrawal symptoms to occur, so it's naturally the most difficult time. But if you find you can put up with mild-to-moderate side effects, don't get discouraged – keep going.

However, as previously advised, if you feel light-headed or dizzy, have a level of headache or muscle pain you rate as severe, or develop a rash you don't think is normal, stop the detox program immediately and see your doctor. Otherwise, any unpleasant side effects will eventually settle down.

HOMEMADE FACIALS

YOGURT AND HONEY CLEANSER

1 tablespoon honey
¼ cup (70g) natural yogurt
rose essential oil

1. Combine honey and yogurt in small bowl. Add a few drops of rose essential oil; mix well.
2. Apply cleanser generously to damp face; massage into skin in an upward circular motion, avoiding eye area. Remove cleanser from face using warm face washer. Rinse face with warm water; pat dry.
TIP: Store remaining cleanser in a screw-top jar in the refrigerator for one week.

KIWI FRUIT AND LIME TONER

2 medium kiwi fruit (170g), peeled, chopped coarsely
⅓ cup (80ml) fresh lime juice

1. Using a food processor, process kiwi fruit until almost smooth; transfer to small bowl, add lime juice, mix well.
2. Place a new piece of muslin, in a single layer, in small strainer over a bowl. Pour fruit mixture over muslin cloth; using a rubber spatula, gently push liquid through cloth and strainer. Discard pulp and seeds.
3. Using a cotton ball, apply toner to face after cleansing, avoiding eye area. Rinse face with cool water; pat dry.
TIP: Store remaining toner in a screw-top jar in refrigerator for one week.

ALMOND AND PAPAYA FACIAL SCRUB

¼ cup (40g) blanched almonds
⅓ cup (40g) oat bran
1 teaspoon sweet almond oil
2 tablespoons pureed papaya flesh
1 tablespoon natural yogurt
2 tablespoons honey

1. Using a food processor, process almonds until they resemble fine breadcrumbs; transfer to small bowl. Add remaining ingredients, mix well.
2. Apply small amount of scrub to damp cleansed face. Gently rub in a circular motion over face concentrating on problem areas, avoid eye area. Rinse face with warm water; pat dry.
TIP: Store remaining scrub in a screw-top jar in refrigerator for one week.

MOISTURISING APRICOT AND ALMOND MASK

½ cup (75g) dried apricots
1 cup (250ml) hot water
1 tablespoon skim milk powder
2 tablespoons sweet almond oil
1 tablespoon hot water, extra

1. Combine apricots and the water in small bowl; soak for 20 minutes or until apricots are softened. Drain.
2. Using a food processor, process apricots with remaining ingredients until smooth.
3. Apply mask, using a small spatula, to clean, dry face, avoiding eye and lip area. Relax for 15 minutes. Remove mask with a warm face washer; rinse and pat dry.

BANANA AND AVOCADO MASK

¼ medium ripe banana (50g)
¼ medium ripe avocado (50g)
1 teaspoon honey
3 teaspoons cornflour

1. Using a fork, mash banana and avocado in a small bowl until almost smooth. Push mixture through a small sieve using the back of a spoon into a small bowl. Add honey and cornflour; mix well.
2. Apply mask, using a small spatula, to a clean, dry face, avoiding eye and lip area. Relax for 15 minutes. Remove mask with a warm face washer; rinse and pat dry.

CUCUMBER, STRAWBERRY AND GRAPE COOLING MASK

20 small seedless red grapes (65g)
½ medium cucumber (85g), seeded, chopped coarsely
3 strawberries (75g), halved
1 tablespoon natural yogurt
½ teaspoon honey

1. Using a food processor, process grapes, cucumber and strawberry until combined.
2. Place a large, new piece of muslin, folded in quarters, in small bowl. Spoon mixture into centre of cloth; gather corners of cloth and twist to squeeze liquid from mixture into bowl; discard liquid. Place fruit pulp into cleaned small bowl. Add yogurt and honey; mix well.
3. Apply mask, using a small spatula, to a clean, dry face, avoiding eye and lip area. Relax for 15 minutes. Gently remove mask with a warm face washer; rinse with warm water and pat dry.

Remember, it's about self-pampering, something to gradually build into your life even after you finish your detox program.

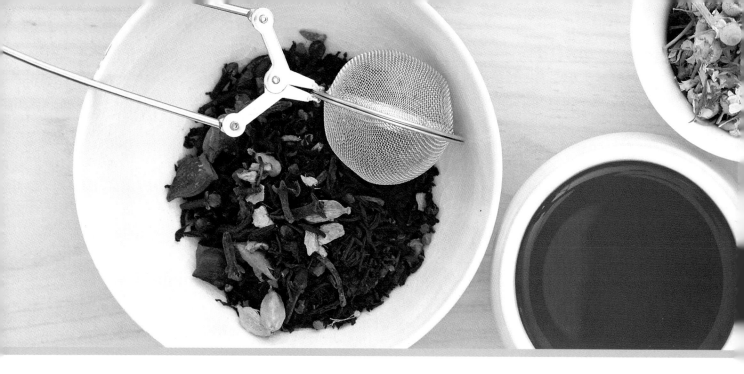

HERBAL TEAS

Herbal teas are no longer the brew of choice only for health fanatics or those who are vehemently anti-caffeine. These calming, reviving and healing teas have become more mainstream as an ever-increasing number of people discover their exotic flavours and soothing medicinal qualities.

The result is that it is easier than ever to order a herbal tea at a chic cafe, or to buy some – not just at specialised tea shops or health-food stores, but also in supermarkets.

There are literally hundreds of different blends you can experiment with – if you do buy your tea from a specialist shop, ask the staff to suggest something to suit your tastes and needs.

Meanwhile, here are a few suggestions to get you started:

- If you're looking for a vitamin C boost, brew yourself some rosehip tea. Vitamin C can help strengthen your immune system and it's also vital for anti-ageing.
- Raspberry tea is also a good source of vitamin C. It can be used as a blood purifier and tonic as well as help control diarrhoea. It can also help in reducing painful menstruation.
- Strawberry leaf tea is believed to help soothe stomach troubles and eczema.
- Tea made with thyme can help improve your immune system as well as promote perspiration, both ideal during a detox.
- After dinner, a peppermint tea can

> **Get rid of negative emotions; laugh more, be more patient, talk about your emotions rather than bottle them up.**

stimulate digestion, while camomile tea helps soothe the stomach and nerves to prepare you for a good night's sleep.

- Dandelion tea is an effective diuretic that can also help improve liver function.
- Lemon balm tea can help lift your spirits.
- Teas containing chaparral, schisandra and St Mary's thistle are all potent ways to treat toxic poisoning of the body. Therefore, they're a great detox tool.

Look for these herbs in tea blends and, for maximum detoxing properties, choose high quality loose-leaf teas, not tea bags.

You need to steep the tea in boiling water for at least three minutes to gain benefits from its healing properties.

Buying yourself a beautiful teapot, or cup and saucer, can help turn brewing a pot of herbal tea into a special ritual.

DETOXING YOUR EMOTIONS

For a detox to work on all aspects of your life, you need to do more than cleanse your body... you need to detox your emotions.

Holistic healers believe that old resentments can burden your body and deplete your energy and, surprisingly, this idea is slowly becoming more accepted by practioners of traditional medicine.

That's because there is increasing evidence that emotions create chemical reactions in the body, and that these substances, which have the potential to cause health problems later, can be stored in muscles and organs.

This area of "emotional" science is called neuroscience or "bodymind" medicine. While much more research is needed into the field,

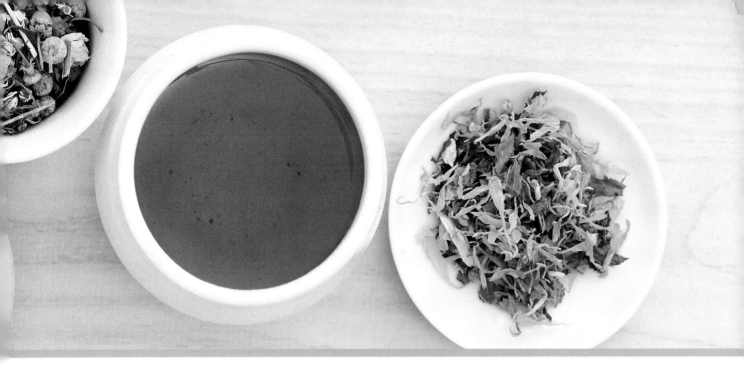

there is no doubt that holding onto anger, resentment, frustration or envy can wear down your mind and body.

If nothing else, you will regularly feel fatigued and have a diminished capacity to enjoy your everyday life.

Emotional detoxing means not only addressing these old "wounds", but also any harmful thought patterns and habits that lead to fear and anxiety – both of which can impact on your health.

So take some time during your detox program to sit quietly and think about what negative emotions you regularly feel, or what negative thoughts consistently run through your mind.

You may decide that you need to learn to laugh more, to be more patient with others – or yourself – to talk about your emotions rather than bottle them up – or even to give up being a perfectionist.

At the same time, you may want to let go of old hurts or disappointments that prevent you being healthy and happy. It may be a simple matter of forgiving others – or yourself – for what is in the past, or simply accepting something the way it is.

A simple ceremony, such as burning a letter in which you have written the feelings or experiences you want to shed, or spending 20 minutes a day during detox in quiet meditation, may be all the emotional medicine you need.

However, if you discover some deep emotional issues that you think you need help in dealing with, seek the support of a therapist or counsellor after your detox to help you achieve a state of wellness and fulfilment. Remember, one of the aims of a detox is to learn how to look after yourself using healthy food, regular exercise and self-pampering. Practising positive self-talk and addressing toxic emotions should be part of your resolve to stay well.

Why not make it a regular habit to spend 30 minutes a day relaxing and detoxing your mind?

EATING OUT DURING DETOX

If you choose to go to a restaurant while you're detoxing, you probably possess a will of iron. After all, you'll need to avoid the wine list, the dessert menu and many of the entrees or mains that don't fit in with your cleansing program. That said, if you really want to eat out, here are some tips to help you avoid falling off the detox wagon.

First, tell your dining companions that you are on a detox program rather than make excuses about why you're not having a glass of wine, or passing on the tiramisu.

Second, you may need to tell the waiter that you don't want butter, oil or salt added to your food. Choose a salad on the menu, without any dressing, or a vegetarian entree or main. And don't be afraid to ask how the meals have been prepared, or to request that certain ingredients be omitted.

Bottled water is a good drink choice, but you may find that the restaurant is also happy to prepare a fresh juice.

Enjoy the company of friends, rather than concentrating on the food, and you'll find eating out is not as daunting as it sounds.

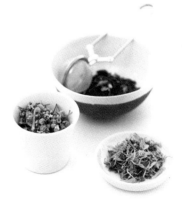

COMING OUT OF DETOX

It's important to ease your body out of a detox program. That's why we've included a "day after" menu in the one-week and two-week detoxes. After you've gone through these menus, continue on the straight and narrow with a healthy, varied diet based on the key foods found in the detoxing menus.

Try not to over-exert yourself and, if possible, don't rush straight back to anything that will cause you stress. Don't be surprised if you feel different emotionally as well as physically – remember, you've cleared out toxins that have been weighing down your body and mind.

AFTER DETOX

In a perfect world, everyone who goes on a detox would continue to live a lifestyle that was so healthy they'd never need to detox again. But we live in the real world, with all its physical, mental and emotional challenges and temptations, so that's just not possible. What we can aim for is to take some of the healthy dietary habits we learned during our detox into our everyday life and add relaxation and exercise programs that keep our body and mind healthy.

Keep your pantry and fridge stocked with the natural, energy-giving foods you enjoyed on your detox. Buy in-season fruit and vegetables to get maximum nutritional benefit and, if possible, buy organic.

> **Ideally, everyone who goes on a detox would continue to live an idyllic lifestyle that was so healthy they'd never need to detox again.**

Remember, stress is one of the major contributors to a toxic state of health, so build pampering and healing routines into your daily life as well. And don't forget to spend some time each day detoxing negative emotions.

After your detox, we strongly recommend you begin and maintain a regular exercise program. Exercise improves circulation, so your body can carry oxygen and expel wastes more effectively; enhances your sense of wellbeing; helps control your appetite and your weight; and de-stresses your body. Without exercise the adrenalin you produce in a hyperactive state has no outlet and can harm muscles, joints and organs.

You don't need to pound the pavements. While you're detoxing, make a plan to learn Pilates, yoga, tai chi or other gentle forms of exercise that treat the body and the mind. Other ideas for fun exercise include hiking, abseiling, trampolining, rollerblading, skiing, cycling and dancing.

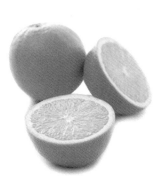

MORE WAYS TO REDUCE TOXIC OVERLOAD

● Avoid using plastics in food preparation. Store food in glass containers and use greaseproof paper instead of plastic wrap.

● Use stainless steel, glass or earthenware in the kitchen and avoid containers made with aluminium and copper, because they can leach metals into foods.

● Keep chemicals in and around your house, garden and car to a minimum. Replace chemical sprays and cleaners with hot water and natural products such as washing soda, borax or bicarbonate of soda. Olive oil makes a good furniture polish.

● Spring-clean your home and donate any clothes, ornaments or pictures you don't really need to charity.

● Avoid anything that is bleached with chlorine, including coffee filter paper and tea bags that don't say they're unbleached. These can contain minute amounts of highly toxic dioxins.

● Avoid walking in highly polluted parts of the city, and always wear a mask if you cycle through city streets.

● Use a water filter to remove chlorine, or buy pure bottled water.

● Use medication, including painkillers, only if absolutely necessary.

● If you must drink, choose a spirit. Although beer and wine have a lower percentage of alcohol, they contain fermentative wastes that are highly acid-forming and toxic to tissues. To make matters worse, most contain chemical contaminants such as preservatives, artificial dyes and other toxic additives.

● Try not to sit in front of a computer for more than five hours a day. Research suggests even low-level radiation for long periods may place the body under toxic stress. Turn off your computer when you're sitting at your desk, but not using it. Get away from it completely by going for a walk at lunchtime.

● Invest in houseplants such as ferns, palms and chrysanthemums as they help reduce levels of chemicals. Take a small pot plant to work and place it on your desk to help reduce pollutants from photocopiers, computers and printers.

● Eat enzyme-rich foods, such as pineapple and sprouted foods, to encourage proper digestion and elimination. Take an enzyme supplement, available at health-food stores, if you have been on antibiotics, or suffer from poor digestion.

● Always wash any fruit and vegetables.

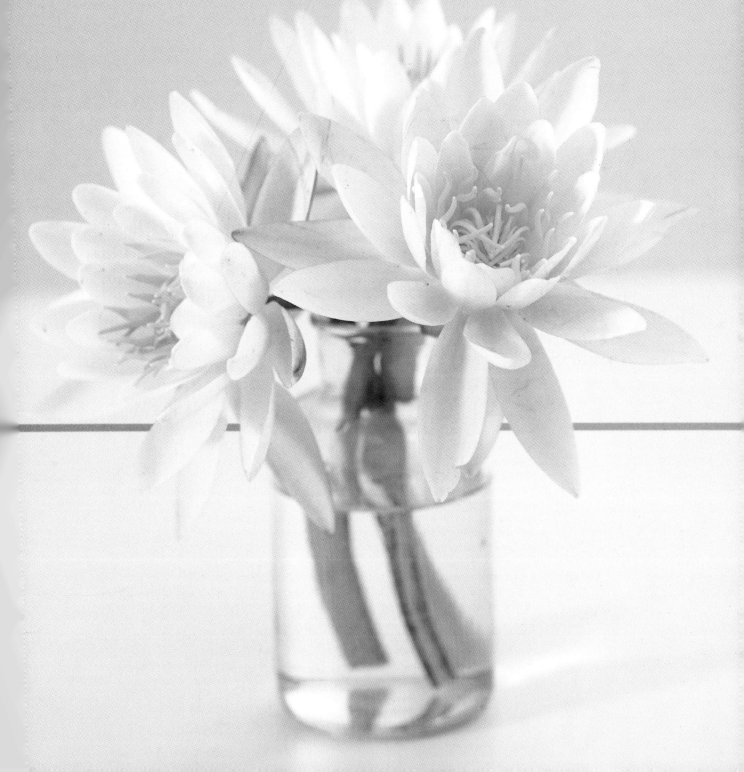

What we can aim for is to take some of the healthy dietary habits we learned during our detox into our everyday life, and add relaxation and exercise programs to keep our body and mind healthy.

menu plans

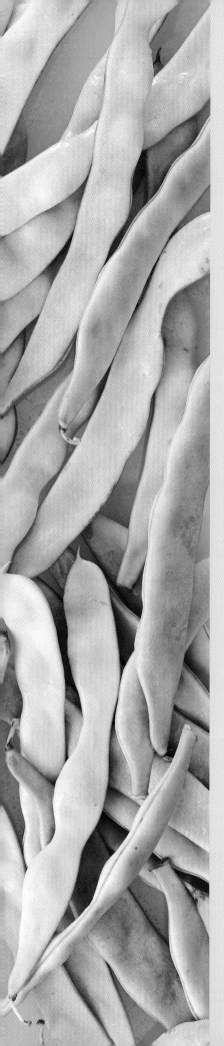

one-day mono-food detox

This can be a good way to introduce yourself to the idea of detox. It's simple: you just eat one type of raw fruit or vegetable for the entire day. The food most commonly chosen is grapes, but you may also like to consider apples, pears, carrots or even papaya.

Make sure you eat lightly the night before your one-day detox, and get plenty of rest.

Breakfast
Hot lemon water *page 112*
Grapes or grape juice (or your chosen fruit or vegetable)

Morning Tea
Grapes or grape juice (or your chosen fruit or vegetable)
Filtered water

Lunch
Grapes or grape juice (or your chosen fruit or vegetable)
Filtered water

Afternoon Tea
Grapes or grape juice (or your chosen fruit or vegetable)
Herbal tea *page 16*

Dinner
Grapes or grape juice (or your chosen fruit or vegetable)
Filtered water or herbal tea *page 16*

Don't go mad the next day – ease out of your detox gently with a light, healthy diet.

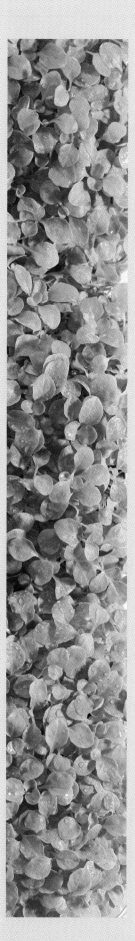

one weekend detox

THE NIGHT BEFORE
Dinner
Mixed bean salad *page 31*

DAY ONE
Breakfast
Hot lemon water *page 112*
Peach, apple and strawberry juice *page 40*
Papaya with passionfruit and lime *page 107*

Morning tea
Watermelon and mint juice *page 43*

Lunch
Lamb's lettuce salad with pecans and orange *page 81*

Afternoon tea
Watercress, beetroot and celery juice *page 40*

Dinner
Asian broth *page 52*

DAY TWO
Breakfast
Hot lemon water *page 112*
Orange and ginger juice *page 42*
Mango cheeks with lime wedges *page 111*

Morning tea
Pineapple, orange and strawberry juice *page 43*

Lunch
Green vegetable salad with american mustard dressing *page 78*

Afternoon tea
Ginger tea *page 115*

Dinner
Stir-fried asian greens with tofu *page 60*

NOTE: Juices should be no larger than 250ml. You should always rinse your mouth or clean your teeth after drinking citrus juices as they're acid and could damage your teeth enamel.

seven-day detox

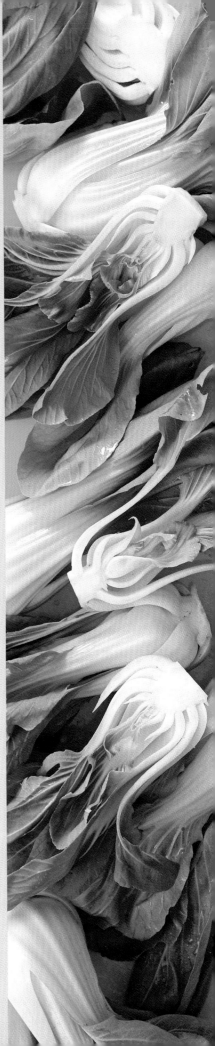

THE DAY BEFORE

Breakfast
Apple and blueberry muesli *page 32*

Lunch
White bean salad *page 27*

Dinner
Vegetable stir-fry served with
steamed brown rice *page 33*

DAY ONE

Breakfast
Hot lemon water *page 112*
Mixed berry juice *page 42*
Four-fruit combo *page 106*

Morning tea
Watermelon and mint juice *page 43*

Lunch
Orange, fennel and almond
salad *page 82*

Afternoon tea
Beetroot, carrot and spinach
juice *page 43*

Dinner
Roasted cherry tomatoes, broccolini
and pepitas *page 62*

DAY TWO

Breakfast
Hot lemon water *page 112*
Strawberry and papaya juice *page 40*
1 banana

Morning tea
Mixed berry juice *page 42*

Lunch
Spinach and zucchini salad
with yogurt hummus *page 83*

Afternoon tea
Grapes

Dinner
Ratatouille *page 63*

DAY THREE

Breakfast
Hot lemon water *page 112*
Raspberry and peach juice *page 42*
1 nectarine

Morning tea
Grapes

Lunch
Greek salad *page 84*

Afternoon tea
Silverbeet, apple and celery
juice *page 44*

Dinner
Black-eyed beans with kumara,
shallots and garlic *page 64*

DAY FOUR

Breakfast
Hot lemon water *page 112*
Orange, carrot and ginger
juice *page 49*
Macerated fruits *page 106*

Morning tea
Watercress, beetroot and celery
juice *page 40*

Lunch
Roasted tomato and capsicum
soup *page 53*

Afternoon tea
Strawberry, honey and soy
smoothie *page 44*

Dinner
Stir-fried asian greens with mixed
mushrooms and steamed brown
rice *page 72*

DAY FIVE

Breakfast
Hot lemon water *page 112*
Mango and grapefruit juice *page 44*
Cherries and yogurt *page 111*

Morning tea
½ mango

Lunch
Potato and bean salad with
lemon yogurt dressing *page 85*

Afternoon tea
Mint tea *page 115*

Dinner
Roasted vegetable stack *page 65*

DAY SIX

Breakfast
Hot lemon water *page 112*
Peach, apple and strawberry
juice *page 40*
Apple and blueberry muesli *page 32*

Morning tea
Pineapple, ginger and mint
juice *page 46*

Lunch
Vegetable soup *page 54*
Lamb's lettuce salad with pecans
and orange *page 81*

Afternoon tea
Carrot dip with crudités *page 76*

Dinner
Pearl barley salad *page 88*

DAY SEVEN

Breakfast
Hot lemon water *page 112*
Pear and ginger juice *page 48*
Macerated fruits *page 106*

Morning tea
Orange, carrot and ginger
juice *page 49*

Lunch
Dhal with vegetables *page 66*

Afternoon tea
Beetroot, carrot and spinach
juice *page 43*

Dinner
Pan-fried tofu with vietnamese
coleslaw salad *page 86*

THE DAY AFTER

Breakfast
Apple and blueberry muesli *page 32*

Lunch
Salad, goat cheese and pecan
sandwich *page 28*

Dinner
Steamed asian bream *page 34*

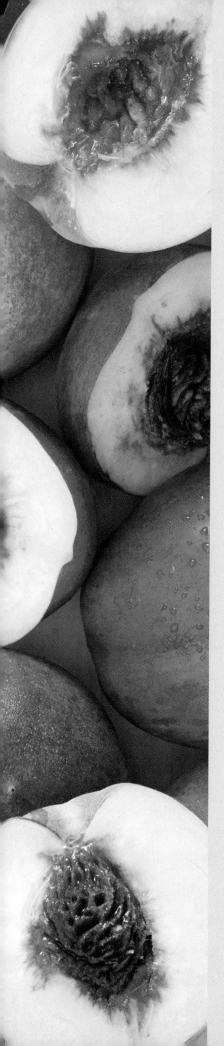

two-week detox

TWO DAYS BEFORE
Breakfast
Apple and pear juice *page 44*
Apple and blueberry muesli *page 32*

Lunch
Open rye sandwich *page 30*

Dinner
Grilled blue-eye with gai larn *page 36*

ONE DAY BEFORE
Breakfast
Pear and ginger juice *page 48*
Apple and blueberry muesli *page 32*

Lunch
Asparagus caesar salad *page 24*

Dinner
Vegetable and white bean
stew *page 37*

DAY ONE   1
Breakfast
Hot lemon water *page 112*
Apple and celery juice *page 45*
Banana with passionfruit
yogurt *page 107*

Morning Tea
Pineapple, ginger and mint
juice *page 46*

Lunch
Greek salad *page 84*

Afternoon Tea
Lemon grass and kaffir lime leaf
tea *page 114*

Dinner
Brown rice with vegetables
and tahini dressing *page 67*

DAY TWO   2
Breakfast
Hot lemon water *page 112*
Mandarin juice *page 46*
Apple and pear compote with
dates *page 104*

Morning Tea
Mint tea *page 115*

Lunch
Cos, snow pea and roasted
celeriac salad *page 89*

Afternoon Tea
Beetroot, carrot and spinach
juice *page 43*

Dinner
Brown rice pilaf *page 75*

DAY THREE   3
Breakfast
Hot lemon water *page 112*
Ginger, orange and pineapple
juice *page 46*
Kiwi fruit, lychee and lime salad
page 108

Morning Tea
Grapes

Lunch
Chickpea, watercress and
capsicum salad *page 90*

Afternoon Tea
Hummus with crudités *page 77*

Dinner
Baked potato with guacamole *page 68*

DAY FOUR   4
Breakfast
Hot lemon water *page 112*
Grapefruit and blood orange
juice *page 47*
1 banana

Morning Tea
Melon slices (one type)

Lunch
Potato and asparagus salad with
yogurt and mint dressing *page 91*

Afternoon Tea
Silverbeet, apple and celery
juice *page 44*

Dinner
Leek, goat cheese and brown
lentil bake *page 69*

DAY FIVE   5
Breakfast
Hot lemon water *page 112*
Kiwi fruit and green grape
juice *page 47*
Figs and sheep milk yogurt
and honey *page 108*

Morning Tea
Pineapple, orange and strawberry
juice *page 43*

Lunch
Borlotti bean, brown rice and
almond salad *page 93*

Afternoon Tea
Cardamom and chamomile
tea *page 114*

Dinner
Roasted egg tomatoes with barley
salad *page 94*

DAY SIX   6
Breakfast
Hot lemon water *page 112*
Apple and pear juice *page 44*
Banana with passionfruit *page 109*

Morning Tea
Strawberry, honey and soy
smoothie *page 44*

Lunch
Pear, spinach, walnut and
celery salad *page 95*

Afternoon Tea
Beetroot dip with crudités *page 76*

Dinner
Roasted root vegetables with
yogurt *page 70*

DAY SEVEN   7
Breakfast
Hot lemon water *page 112*
Orange, carrot and celery juice *page 48*
Apple and pear compote with
dates *page 104*

Morning Tea
Tangelo and ginger juice *page 47*

Lunch
Leek and potato soup *page 55*

Afternoon Tea
Cinnamon and orange tea *page 115*

Dinner
Brown rice with vegetables and
tahini dressing *page 67*

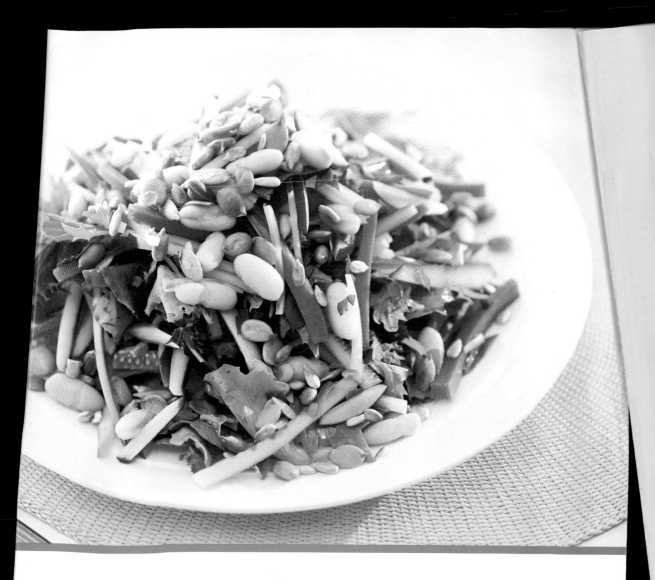

PORRIDGE WITH POACHED PEARS AND BLUEBERRIES

PREPARATION TIME **10 MINUTES** COOKING TIME **10 MINUTES** SERVES 1

ERVING
OTAL FAT
(SATURATED FAT)
CARBOHYDRATE
(211 CAL)
PROTEIN
FIBRE

¾ cup (180ml) hot water
⅓ cup (30g) rolled oats
1 small pear (180g), cored, chopped coarsely
½ cup (125ml) cold water
2 tablespoons frozen blueberries, thawed

1 Combine the hot water and oats in small saucepan over medium heat; cook, stirring, about 5 minutes or until porridge is thick and creamy.
2 Meanwhile, place pear and the cold water in small saucepan; bring to a boil. Reduce heat; simmer, uncovered, about 5 minutes or until pear has softened.
3 Serve porridge topped with pears and 1 tablespoon of the poaching liquid; sprinkle with berries.

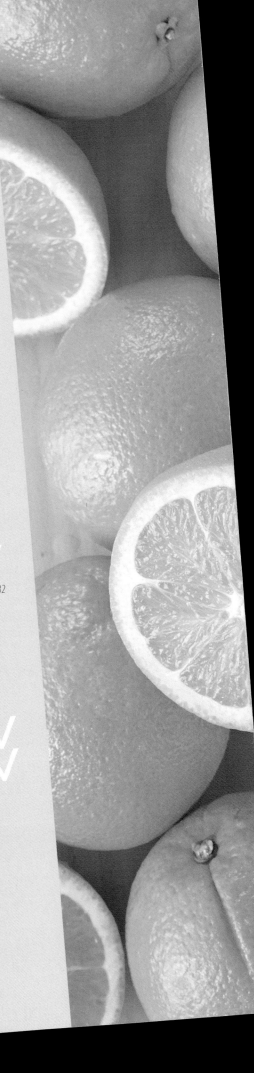

DAY EIGHT 8
Breakfast
Hot lemon water *page 112*
Mandarin juice *page 46*
1 pear

Morning Tea
1 custard apple

Lunch
Eggplant with salsa fresca *page 71*

Afternoon Tea
Raita with crudités *page 77*

Dinner
Thai soy bean salad with grapes and pink grapefruit *page 96*

DAY NINE 9
Breakfast
Hot lemon water *page 112*
Ginger, orange and pineapple juice *page 46*
Lychees with passionfruit *page 109*

Morning Tea
Blood plums with honey and cardamom yogurt *page 110*

Lunch
Soba salad with seaweed, ginger and vegetables *page 98*

Afternoon Tea
Mint tea *page 115*

Dinner
Grilled asparagus with warm tomato dressing *page 97*

DAY TEN 10
Breakfast
Hot lemon water *page 112*
Pear and grape juice *page 45*
Stewed prunes with orange *page 110*

Morning Tea
Lemon grass and kaffir lime leaf tea *page 114*

Lunch
Pumpkin and kumara soup *page 56*

Afternoon Tea
Carrot dip with crudités *page 76*

Dinner
Baked beetroot salad with cannellini beans, fetta and mint *page 103*

DAY ELEVEN 11
Breakfast
Hot lemon water *page 112*
Orange, carrot and celery juice *page 48*
Mango cheeks with lime wedges *page 111*

Morning Tea
1 banana

Lunch
Roasted pumpkin, pecan and fetta salad *page 101*

Afternoon Tea
Ginger tea *page 115*

Dinner
Stir-fried asian greens with mixed mushrooms *page 72*

DAY TWELVE 12
Breakfast
Hot lemon water *page 112*
Orange, mango and strawberry juice *page 48*
1 cup mixed berries

Morning Tea
Watercress, beetroot and celery juice *page 40*

Lunch
Vegetable and soba soup *page 57*

Afternoon Tea
Beetroot dip and crudités *page 76*

Dinner
Chickpea patties with tomato and cucumber salad *page 73*

DAY THIRTEEN 13
Breakfast
Hot lemon water *page 112*
Orange, carrot and ginger juice *page 49*
Watermelon slices

Morning Tea
Cinnamon and orange tea *page 115*

Lunch
Dhal with vegetables *page 66*

Afternoon Tea
Carrot, ginger and silverbeet juice *page 49*

Dinner
Stir-fried tofu with vegetables and lemon grass *page 74*

DAY FOURTEEN 14
Breakfast
Hot lemon water *page 112*
Apple and blueberry museli *page 32*
Melon slices

Morning Tea
Banana soy smoothie *page 49*

Lunch
Tomato and avocado salad with tofu pesto *page 100*

Afternoon Tea
Hummus with crudités *page 77*

Dinner
Lentil and vegetable soup *page 59*

THE DAY AFTER ∨
Breakfast
Apple and blueberry muesli *page 32*

Lunch
Lavash wrap *page 29*

Dinner
Oven-roasted ratatouille with almond gremolata *page 39*

TWO DAYS AFTER ∨
Breakfast
Porridge with poached pears and blueberries *page 26*

Lunch
Vegetable soup *page 54*
Cos, snow pea and roasted celeriac salad *page 89*

Dinner
Poached flathead with herb salad *page 35*

before & after detox

PER SERVING
9g TOTAL FAT
(0.8g SATURATED FAT)
19.7g CARBOHYDRATE
865kJ (207 CAL)
10.2g PROTEIN
6.7g FIBRE

ASPARAGUS CAESAR SALAD

PREPARATION TIME **15 MINUTES** COOKING TIME **10 MINUTES** SERVES **1**

1 slice wholemeal bread (45g), crust removed

1 teaspoon olive oil

½ clove garlic, crushed

170g asparagus, trimmed, chopped coarsely

½ baby cos lettuce (90g), leaves separated

CAESAR DRESSING
½ clove garlic, crushed

1 teaspoon american mustard

2 teaspoons lemon juice

2 tablespoons sheep milk yogurt

1 tablespoon water

1 Preheat oven to moderate (180°C/160°C fan-forced).
2 Cut bread into 3cm cubes. Combine oil and garlic in small bowl, add bread; toss bread
to coat in mixture. Place bread, in single layer, on oven tray; toast, uncovered, 10 minutes.
3 Meanwhile, place ingredients for caesar dressing in screw-top jar; shake well.
4 Boil, steam or microwave asparagus until just tender; drain.
5 Place croutons and asparagus in medium bowl with lettuce; toss gently to combine.
6 Serve salad drizzled with dressing.

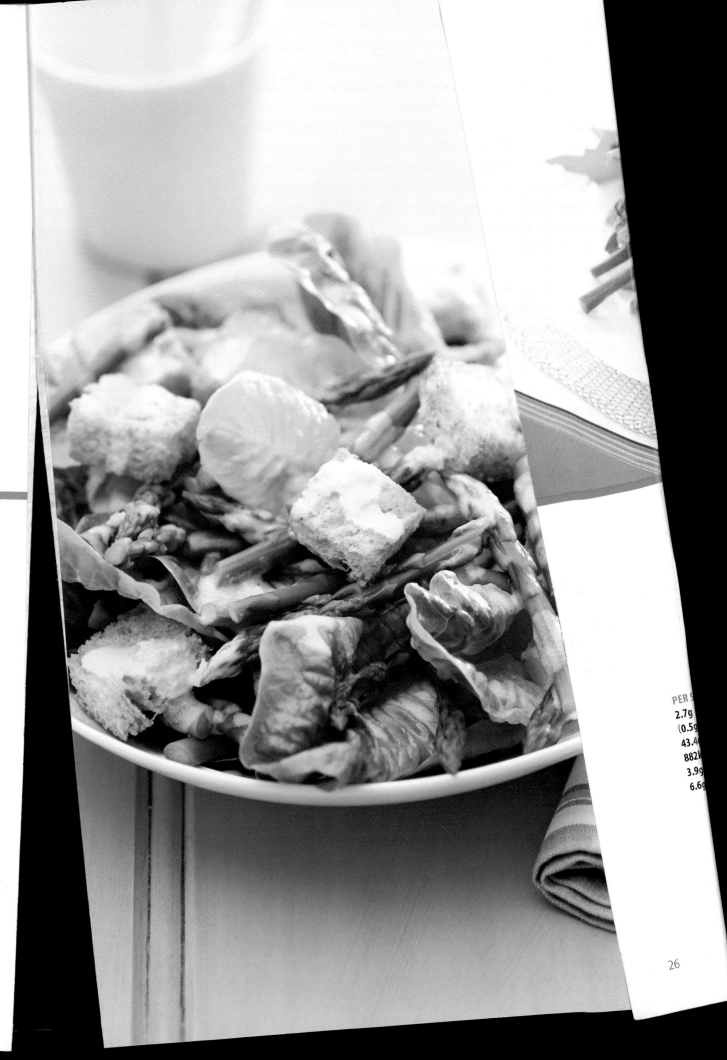

PER S
2.7g
(0.5g
43.4
882k
3.9g
6.6g

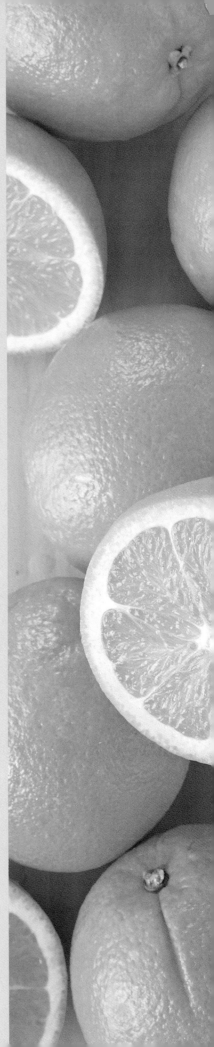

DAY EIGHT
Breakfast
Hot lemon water *page 112*
Mandarin juice *page 46*
1 pear

Morning Tea
1 custard apple

Lunch
Eggplant with salsa fresca *page 71*

Afternoon Tea
Raita with crudités *page 77*

Dinner
Thai soy bean salad with grapes
and pink grapefruit *page 96*

DAY NINE
Breakfast
Hot lemon water *page 112*
Ginger, orange and pineapple
juice *page 46*
Lychees with passionfruit *page 109*

Morning Tea
Blood plums with honey and
cardamom yogurt *page 110*

Lunch
Soba salad with seaweed, ginger
and vegetables *page 98*

Afternoon Tea
Mint tea *page 115*

Dinner
Grilled asparagus with warm
tomato dressing *page 97*

DAY TEN
Breakfast
Hot lemon water *page 112*
Pear and grape juice *page 45*
Stewed prunes with orange *page 110*

Morning Tea
Lemon grass and kaffir lime leaf
tea *page 114*

Lunch
Pumpkin and kumara soup *page 56*

Afternoon Tea
Carrot dip with crudités *page 76*

8

Dinner
Baked beetroot salad with cannellini
beans, fetta and mint *page 103*

DAY ELEVEN
Breakfast
Hot lemon water *page 112*
Orange, carrot and celery juice *page 48*
Mango cheeks with lime
wedges *page 111*

Morning Tea
1 banana

Lunch
Roasted pumpkin, pecan and fetta
salad *page 101*

Afternoon Tea
Ginger tea *page 115*

Dinner
Stir-fried asian greens with
mixed mushrooms *page 72*

DAY TWELVE
Breakfast
Hot lemon water *page 112*
Orange, mango and strawberry
juice *page 48*
1 cup mixed berries

Morning Tea
Watercress, beetroot and celery
juice *page 40*

Lunch
Vegetable and soba soup *page 57*

Afternoon Tea
Beetroot dip and crudités *page 76*

Dinner
Chickpea patties with tomato and
cucumber salad *page 73*

DAY THIRTEEN
Breakfast
Hot lemon water *page 112*
Orange, carrot and ginger
juice *page 49*
Watermelon slices

Morning Tea
Cinnamon and orange tea *page 115*

11

12

13

9

10

Lunch
Dhal with vegetables *page 66*

Afternoon Tea
Carrot, ginger and silverbeet
juice *page 49*

Dinner
Stir-fried tofu with vegetables
and lemon grass *page 74*

DAY FOURTEEN
Breakfast
Hot lemon water *page 112*
Apple and blueberry museli *page 32*
Melon slices

Morning Tea
Banana soy smoothie *page 49*

Lunch
Tomato and avocado salad
with tofu pesto *page 100*

Afternoon Tea
Hummus with crudités *page 77*

Dinner
Lentil and vegetable soup *page 59*

THE DAY AFTER
Breakfast
Apple and blueberry muesli *page 32*

Lunch
Lavash wrap *page 29*

Dinner
Oven-roasted ratatouille with
almond gremolata *page 39*

TWO DAYS AFTER
Breakfast
Porridge with poached pears
and blueberries *page 26*

Lunch
Vegetable soup *page 54*
Cos, snow pea and roasted
celeriac salad *page 89*

Dinner
Poached flathead with
herb salad *page 35*

14

before & after detox

PER SERVING
9g TOTAL FAT
(0.8g SATURATED FAT)
19.7g CARBOHYDRATE
865kJ (207 CAL)
10.2g PROTEIN
6.7g FIBRE

ASPARAGUS CAESAR SALAD

PREPARATION TIME **15 MINUTES** COOKING TIME **10 MINUTES** SERVES **1**

1 slice wholemeal bread (45g), crust removed

1 teaspoon olive oil

½ clove garlic, crushed

170g asparagus, trimmed, chopped coarsely

½ baby cos lettuce (90g), leaves separated

CAESAR DRESSING
½ clove garlic, crushed

1 teaspoon american mustard

2 teaspoons lemon juice

2 tablespoons sheep milk yogurt

1 tablespoon water

1 Preheat oven to moderate (180°C/160°C fan-forced).
2 Cut bread into 3cm cubes. Combine oil and garlic in small bowl, add bread; toss bread
   to coat in mixture. Place bread, in single layer, on oven tray; toast, uncovered, 10 minutes.
3 Meanwhile, place ingredients for caesar dressing in screw-top jar; shake well.
4 Boil, steam or microwave asparagus until just tender; drain.
5 Place croutons and asparagus in medium bowl with lettuce; toss gently to combine.
6 Serve salad drizzled with dressing.

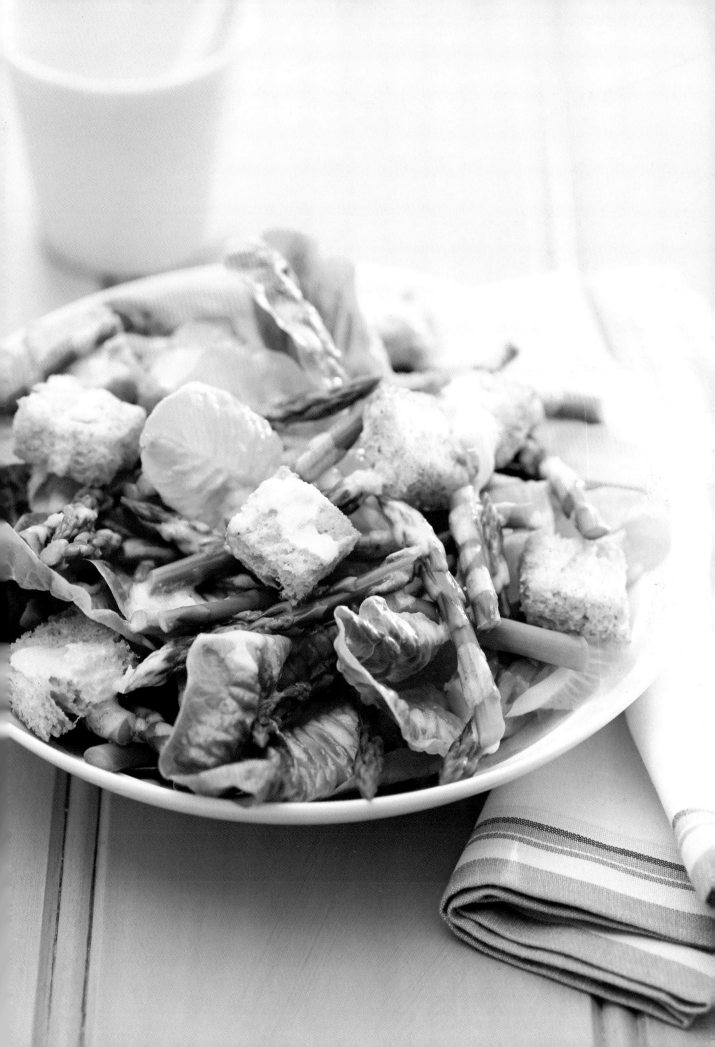

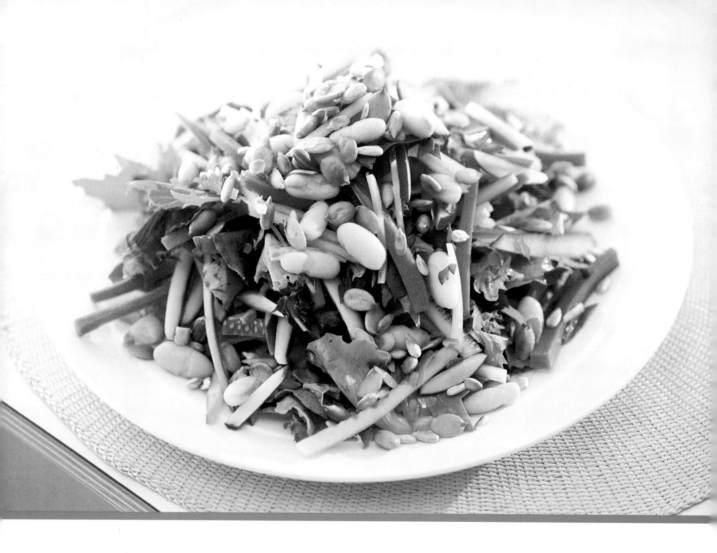

PORRIDGE WITH POACHED PEARS
AND BLUEBERRIES

PREPARATION TIME **10 MINUTES** COOKING TIME **10 MINUTES** SERVES **1**

PER SERVING
2.7g TOTAL FAT
(0.5g SATURATED FAT)
43.4g CARBOHYDRATE
882kJ (211 CAL)
3.9g PROTEIN
6.6g FIBRE

¾ cup (180ml) hot water

⅓ cup (30g) rolled oats

1 small pear (180g), cored, chopped coarsely

½ cup (125ml) cold water

2 tablespoons frozen blueberries, thawed

1 Combine the hot water and oats in small saucepan over medium heat; cook, stirring, about
  5 minutes or until porridge is thick and creamy.
2 Meanwhile, place pear and the cold water in small saucepan; bring to a boil. Reduce heat;
  simmer, uncovered, about 5 minutes or until pear has softened.
3 Serve porridge topped with pears and 1 tablespoon of the poaching liquid; sprinkle with berries.

WHITE BEAN SALAD

PREPARATION TIME **15 MINUTES** SERVES **1**

Many varieties of pre-cooked white beans are available canned, among them cannellini, butter and haricot beans; any of these are suitable for this salad.

50g mesclun

½ cup (100g) canned white beans, rinsed, drained

2 tablespoons coarsely chopped fresh tarragon

2 tablespoons coarsely chopped fresh flat-leaf parsley

1 small carrot (70g), cut into matchsticks

½ lebanese cucumber (65g), cut into matchsticks

2 red radishes (70g), trimmed, cut into matchsticks

2 tablespoons fresh apple juice

1 tablespoon apple cider vinegar

1 tablespoon toasted sunflower seeds

1 tablespoon toasted pepitas

PER SERVING
12.3g TOTAL FAT
(0.5g SATURATED FAT)
21g CARBOHYDRATE
1145kJ (274 CAL)
10.1g PROTEIN
12.5g FIBRE

1 Place mesclun, beans, herbs, carrot, cucumber, radish, juice and vinegar in medium bowl; toss gently to combine.

2 Serve salad topped with seeds.

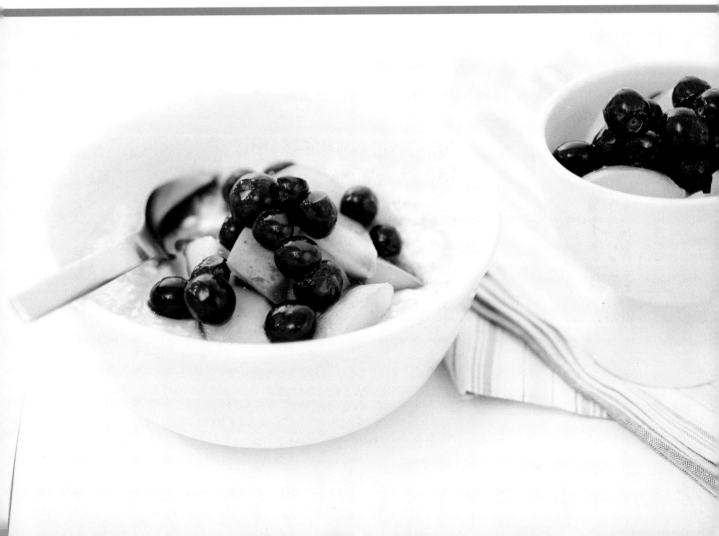

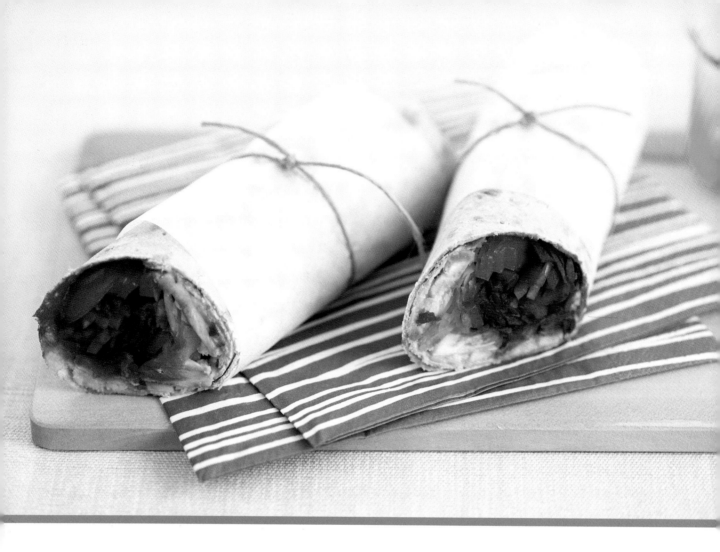

SALAD, GOAT CHEESE AND PECAN SANDWICH

PREPARATION TIME **15 MINUTES** SERVES **1**

PER SERVING
16.5g TOTAL FAT
(**5g** SATURATED FAT)
40.8g CARBOHYDRATE
1593kJ (381 CAL)
17.1g PROTEIN
10.6g FIBRE

40g goat milk cheese

1 tablespoon finely chopped pecans

1 tablespoon coarsely chopped fresh flat-leaf parsley

2 slices wholemeal bread (90g)

1 small tomato (90g), sliced thinly

½ lebanese cucumber (65g), sliced thinly lengthways

½ small carrot (35g), sliced thinly lengthways

2 small baby cos lettuce leaves

1 Combine cheese, nuts and parsley in small bowl.
2 Spread cheese mixture on each slice of bread; top one slice with tomato, cucumber, carrot and lettuce. Top with remaining slice.

LAVASH WRAP

PREPARATION TIME **15 MINUTES** SERVES **1**

1 slice wholemeal lavash

¼ small avocado (50g)

1 teaspoon tahini

½ cup (60g) coarsely grated uncooked beetroot

⅓ cup (50g) coarsely grated uncooked pumpkin

¼ small red capsicum (40g), sliced thinly

40g mushrooms, sliced thinly

¼ small red onion (25g), sliced thinly

PER SERVING
13.4g TOTAL FAT
(2.6g SATURATED FAT)
45.1g CARBOHYDRATE
1463kJ (350 CAL)
12.2g PROTEIN
10.1g FIBRE

1 Spread bread with avocado and tahini.
2 Place remaining ingredients on long side of bread; roll to enclose filling.

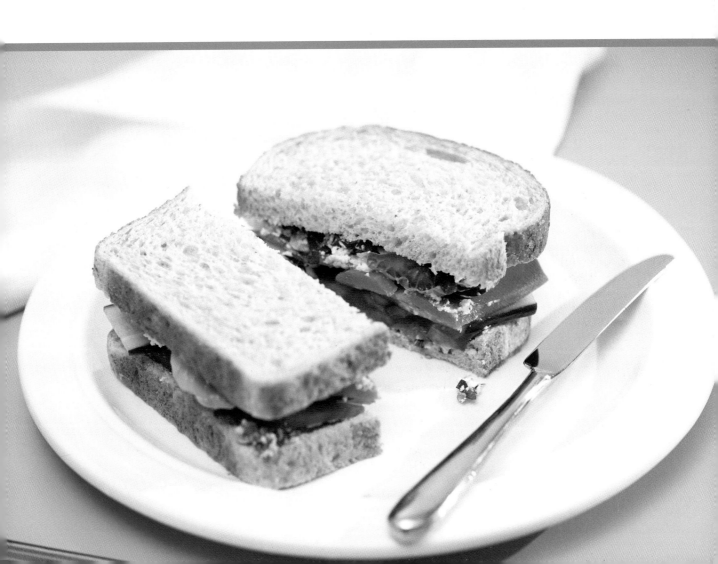

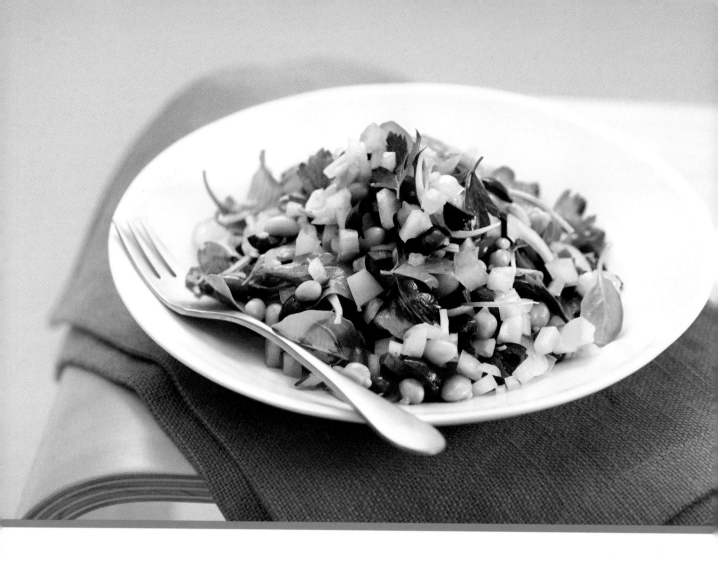

OPEN RYE SANDWICH

PREPARATION TIME **10 MINUTES** SERVES **1**

PER SERVING
3.7g TOTAL FAT
(**1.7g** SATURATED FAT)
21.8g CARBOHYDRATE
635kJ (**152 CAL**)
7.6g PROTEIN
4.9g FIBRE

1 teaspoon finely chopped fresh basil

1 teaspoon finely chopped fresh mint

1 teaspoon finely chopped fresh flat-leaf parsley

1 tablespoon ricotta cheese

1 slice rye bread (40g)

½ cup (10g) loosely packed baby rocket leaves

1 small tomato (90g), sliced thinly

½ lebanese cucumber (65g), sliced thinly

1 tablespoon alfalfa sprouts

1 Combine herbs and cheese in small bowl.

2 Spread cheese mixture on bread; top with remaining ingredients.

MIXED BEAN SALAD

PREPARATION TIME **15 MINUTES** SERVES **1**

1 clove garlic, crushed

2 teaspoons olive oil

2 teaspoons fresh lemon juice

½ x 300g can four-bean mix, rinsed, drained

1 trimmed celery stalk (100g), chopped finely

½ medium yellow capsicum (100g), chopped finely

¼ cup (30g) seeded black olives, chopped coarsely

¼ cup loosely packed fresh flat-leaf parsley leaves

½ small red onion (50g), sliced thinly

1 cup (20g) loosely packed baby rocket leaves

PER SERVING
10.3g TOTAL FAT
(**1.5g** SATURATED FAT)
27.6g CARBOHYDRATE
995kJ (238 CAL)
9.3g PROTEIN
10.5g FIBRE

1 Place garlic, oil and juice in screw-top jar; shake well.
2 Place remaining ingredients and dressing in medium bowl; toss gently to combine.

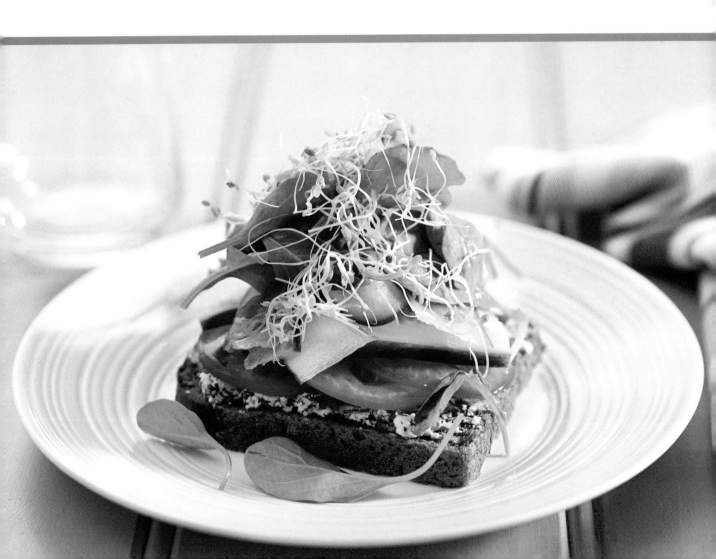

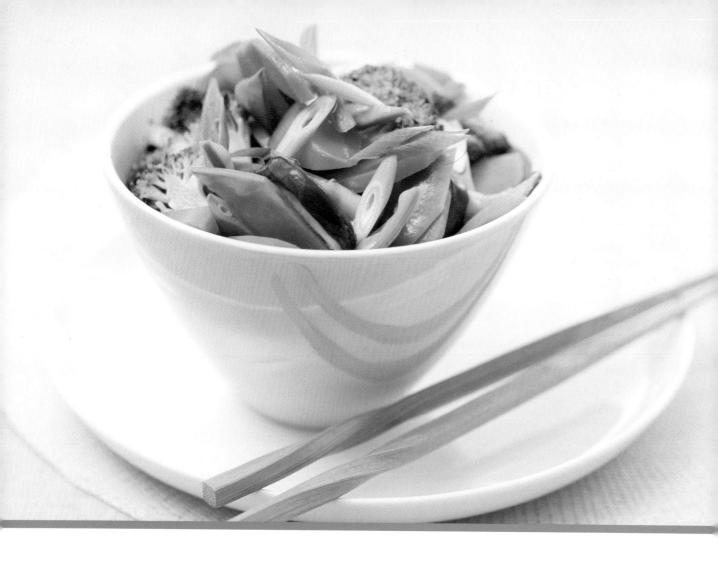

APPLE AND BLUEBERRY MUESLI

PREPARATION TIME **10 MINUTES** (PLUS REFRIGERATION TIME) SERVES **1**

PER SERVING
7.2g TOTAL FAT
(0.2g SATURATED FAT)
39.7g CARBOHYDRATE
1083kJ (259 CAL)
6.7g PROTEIN
3.9g FIBRE

2 tablespoons rolled oats

⅓ cup (80ml) fresh apple juice

½ medium apple (75g), grated coarsely

⅓ cup (50g) blueberries

⅓ cup (95g) sheep milk yogurt

1 tablespoon fresh apple juice, extra

1 tablespoon blueberries, extra

1 Combine oats and juice in small bowl, cover; refrigerate about 1 hour or until oats soften. Stir in apple, blueberries and yogurt.
2 Serve muesli drizzled with extra juice and topped with extra blueberries.

VEGETABLE STIR-FRY

PREPARATION TIME **10 MINUTES** COOKING TIME **10 MINUTES** SERVES **1**

1 teaspoon sesame oil

100g fresh shiitake mushrooms, sliced thickly

1 medium carrot (120g), sliced thinly

2 tablespoons water

100g broccoli, sliced thinly

75g snow peas, trimmed, sliced thickly

1 tablespoon tamari

1 green onion, sliced thinly

PER SERVING
5.4g TOTAL FAT
(0.8g SATURATED FAT)
23.7g CARBOHYDRATE
778kJ (186 CAL)
10.8g PROTEIN
11.7g FIBRE

1 Heat oil in wok; stir-fry mushroom and carrot 2 minutes. Add the water; stir-fry 5 minutes or until carrot just softens. Add broccoli and snow peas; stir-fry until broccoli is just tender. Stir in tamari.

2 Serve stir-fry topped with onion.

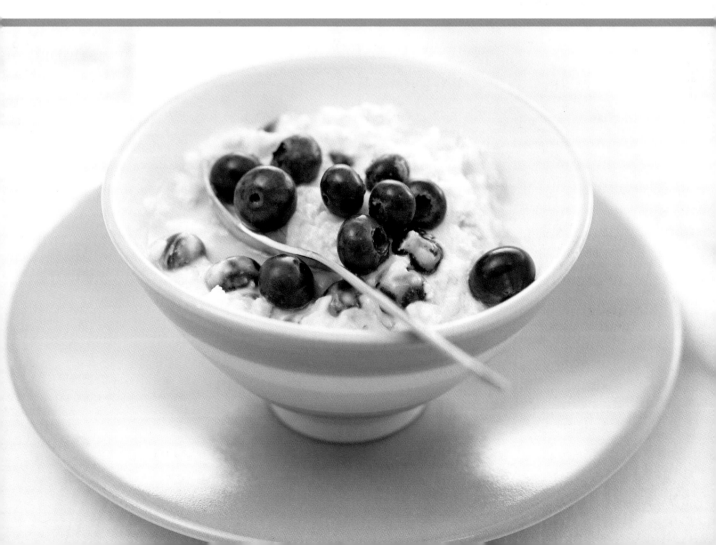

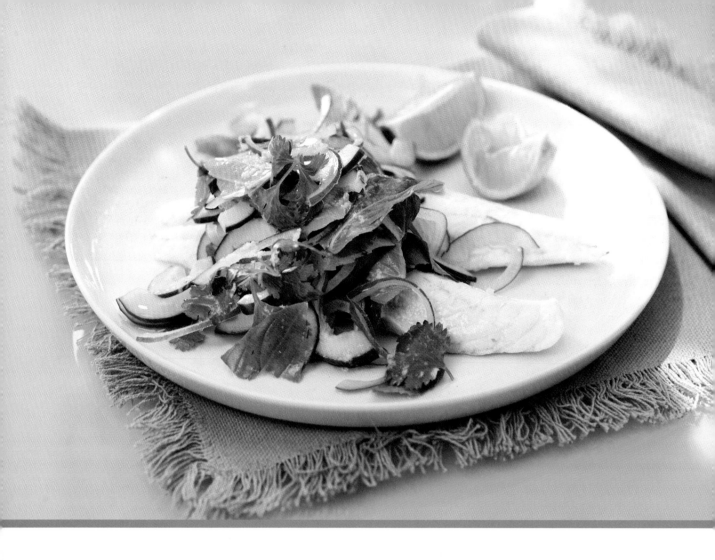

STEAMED ASIAN BREAM

PREPARATION TIME **10 MINUTES** COOKING TIME **15 MINUTES** SERVES **1**

PER SERVING
11.2g TOTAL FAT
(2.9g SATURATED FAT)
5g CARBOHYDRATE
957kJ **(229 CAL)**
26.8g PROTEIN
2.4g FIBRE

1 whole bream (240g)

3cm piece fresh ginger (15g), cut into matchsticks

1 green onion, sliced thinly

1 small carrot (70g), cut into matchsticks

1 tablespoon tamari

1 teaspoon sesame oil

1 Preheat oven to moderately hot (200°C/180°C fan-forced).

2 Lightly oil sheet of foil large enough to enclose fish. Place fish on foil, fill cavity with half of the vegetables. Brush fish with combined tamari and oil; top with remaining vegetables.

3 Fold edges of foil to enclose fish; place fish parcel on oven tray. Cook about 15 minutes or until fish is cooked as desired.

4 Serve fish sprinkled with fresh coriander leaves, if desired.

POACHED FLATHEAD WITH HERB SALAD

PREPARATION TIME **20 MINUTES** COOKING TIME **10 MINUTES** SERVES **1**

3 cups (750ml) water

2 cloves garlic, crushed

5cm piece fresh ginger (25g), sliced thinly

2 flathead fillets (220g)

1 lime, cut into wedges

HERB SALAD

¼ cup loosely packed fresh mint leaves

¼ cup loosely packed fresh coriander leaves

¼ cup loosely packed fresh basil leaves, torn

½ small red onion (50g), sliced thinly

1 lebanese cucumber (130g), seeded, sliced thinly

1 tablespoon fresh lime juice

1cm piece fresh ginger (5g), grated

PER SERVING
3g TOTAL FAT
(**1g** SATURATED FAT)
8.3g CARBOHYDRATE
1124kJ (269 CAL)
49.6g PROTEIN
6.6g FIBRE

1   Place the water, garlic and ginger in medium frying pan; bring to a boil. Add fish, reduce heat; simmer, uncovered, about 5 minutes or until fish is cooked as desired. Remove fish with slotted spoon; discard liquid.

2   Meanwhile, combine ingredients for herb salad in medium bowl.

3   Serve fish with salad and lime wedges.

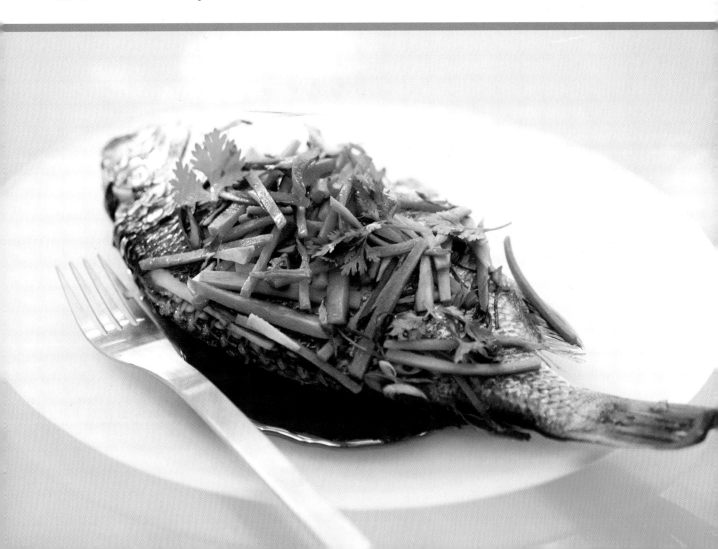

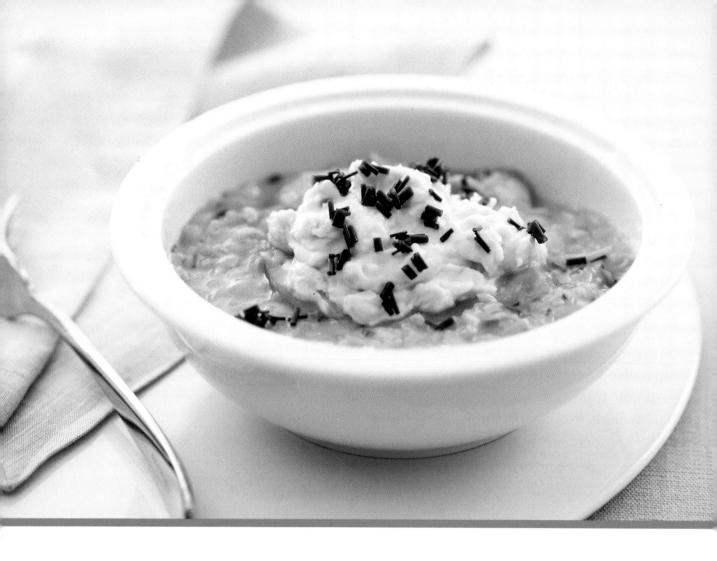

GRILLED BLUE-EYE WITH GAI LARN

PREPARATION TIME **10 MINUTES** COOKING TIME **10 MINUTES** SERVES **1**

PER SERVING
1.7g TOTAL FAT
(0.2g SATURATED FAT)
3.5g CARBOHYDRATE
828kJ (198 CAL)
41.2g PROTEIN
8.2g FIBRE

200g blue-eye fillet

200g gai larn, chopped coarsely

GINGER AND GARLIC DRESSING
2cm piece fresh ginger (10g), grated

1 clove garlic, crushed

1 tablespoon water

1 tablespoon tamari

1 Cook fish in heated lightly oiled small frying pan, uncovered, until cooked through.
2 Meanwhile, boil, steam or microwave gai larn until tender; drain.
3 Place ingredients for ginger and garlic dressing in screw-top jar; shake well.
4 Serve fish with gai larn, drizzle with dressing.

VEGETABLE AND WHITE BEAN STEW

PREPARATION TIME **15 MINUTES** COOKING TIME **30 MINUTES** SERVES **1**

1 teaspoon olive oil

1 small leek (200g), sliced thinly

1 medium carrot (120g), sliced thickly

1 shallot (25g), chopped finely

2 cloves garlic, crushed

2 tablespoons rolled oats

1½ cups (375ml) water

2 tablespoons coarsely chopped fresh chives

½ cup (100g) canned white beans, rinsed, drained

2 teaspoons finely grated lemon rind

2 tablespoons sheep milk yogurt

PER SERVING
9.2g TOTAL FAT
(0.9g SATURATED FAT)
32.9g CARBOHYDRATE
1120kJ **(268 CAL)**
12.7g PROTEIN
13.8g FIBRE

1 Heat oil in medium saucepan; cook leek, carrot, shallot and garlic, stirring, 10 minutes. Add oats and the water; bring to a boil. Reduce heat; simmer, covered, about 15 minutes or until liquid is almost absorbed. Stir in half of the chives.
2 Mash beans with rind and yogurt in small saucepan; cook, stirring, until heated through.
3 Serve stew topped with bean mixture and remaining chives.

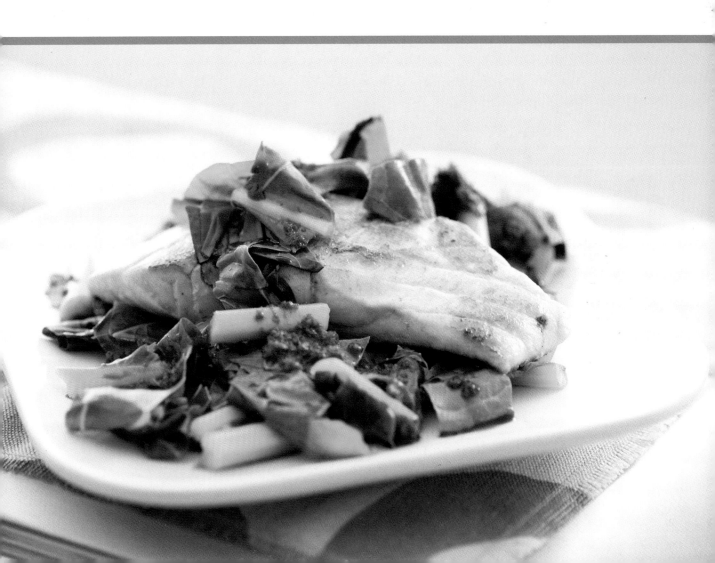

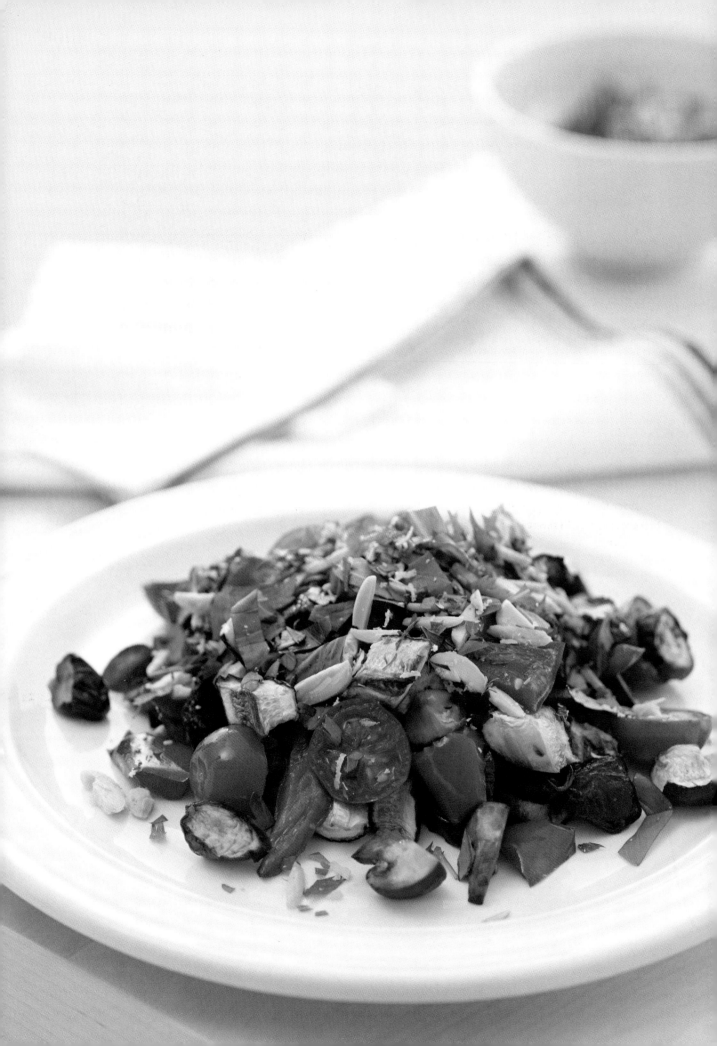

OVEN-ROASTED RATATOUILLE WITH ALMOND GREMOLATA

PREPARATION TIME **10 MINUTES** COOKING TIME **40 MINUTES** SERVES **1**

2 baby eggplants (120g), chopped coarsely

1 medium zucchini (120g), chopped coarsely

1 small red capsicum (150g), chopped coarsely

1 clove garlic, crushed

2 teaspoons olive oil

100g mushrooms, chopped coarsely

125g cherry tomatoes, halved

ALMOND GREMOLATA

2 tablespoons coarsely chopped fresh flat-leaf parsley

2 tablespoons coarsely chopped fresh basil

1 teaspoon finely grated lemon rind

2 tablespoons toasted slivered almonds, chopped coarsely

1 clove garlic, crushed

1 Preheat oven to moderately hot (200°C/180°C fan-forced).
2 Combine eggplant, zucchini, capsicum, garlic and oil in small shallow baking dish. Roast, uncovered, 30 minutes, stirring occasionally. Add mushroom and tomato; roast, uncovered, about 10 minutes or until vegetables are just tender.
3 Meanwhile, combine ingredients for almond gremolata in small bowl.
4 Serve ratatouille topped with gremolata.

PER SERVING
21.6g TOTAL FAT
(**2.4g** SATURATED FAT)
16g CARBOHYDRATE
1304kJ (**312 CAL**)
13.8g PROTEIN
14.2g FIBRE

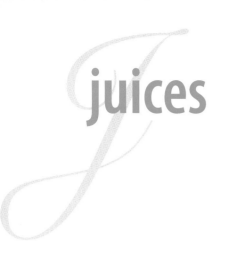

juices

PEACH, APPLE AND STRAWBERRY

We used a green apple in this recipe, but you can use the colour of your choice.

1 medium apple (150g), cut into wedges

1 medium peach (150g), cut into wedges

2 strawberries (40g)

1 Push ingredients through juice extractor into glass; stir to combine.

PER SERVING
0.3g TOTAL FAT
(0g SATURATED FAT)
24.3g CARBOHYDRATE
451kJ (108 CAL)
2.2g PROTEIN
5.1g FIBRE

WATERCRESS, BEETROOT AND CELERY

1 trimmed celery stalk (100g), chopped coarsely

3 baby beetroots (75g), cut into wedges

50g watercress, trimmed

½ cup (125ml) water

1 Push celery, beetroot and watercress through juice extractor into glass.
2 Stir in the water.

PER SERVING
0.4g TOTAL FAT
(0g SATURATED FAT)
8.9g CARBOHYDRATE
222kJ (53 CAL)
3.5g PROTEIN
6g FIBRE

STRAWBERRY AND PAPAYA

We used the red-fleshed Hawaiian or Fijian variety of papaya in this recipe.

4 strawberries (80g)

80g papaya

½ cup (125ml) water

1 Blend or process ingredients until smooth.
   tip For something refreshing, freeze the juice until almost set then scrape with a fork for a granita-like snack.

PER SERVING
0.2g TOTAL FAT
(0g SATURATED FAT)
7.7g CARBOHYDRATE
163kJ (39 CAL)
1.7g PROTEIN
3.6g FIBRE

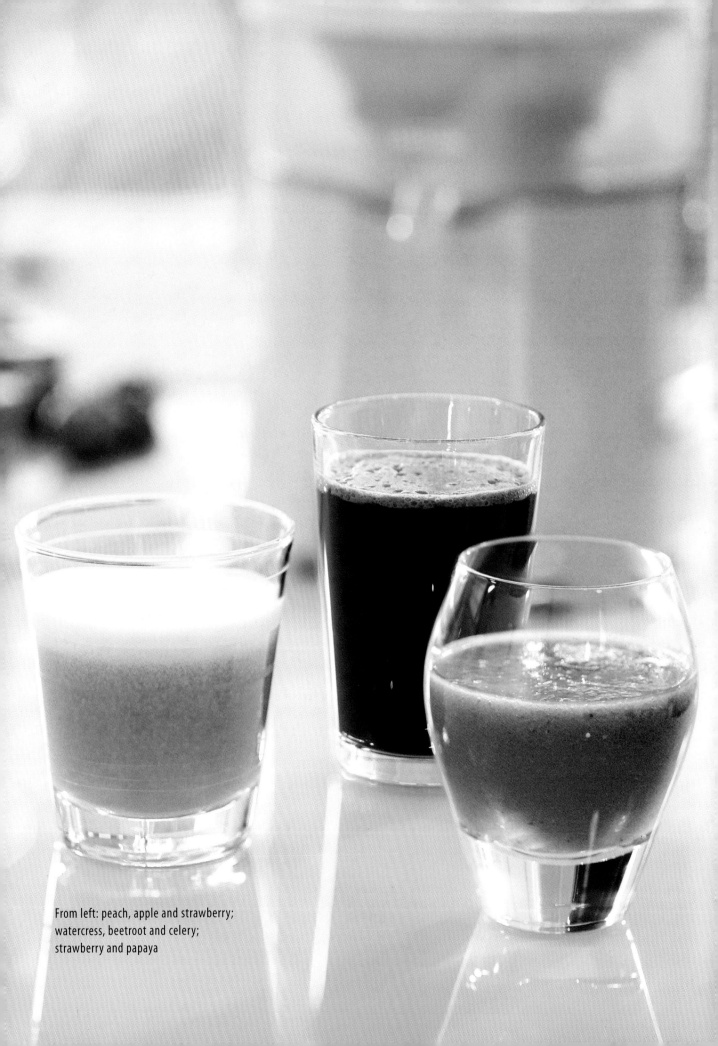

From left: peach, apple and strawberry;
watercress, beetroot and celery;
strawberry and papaya

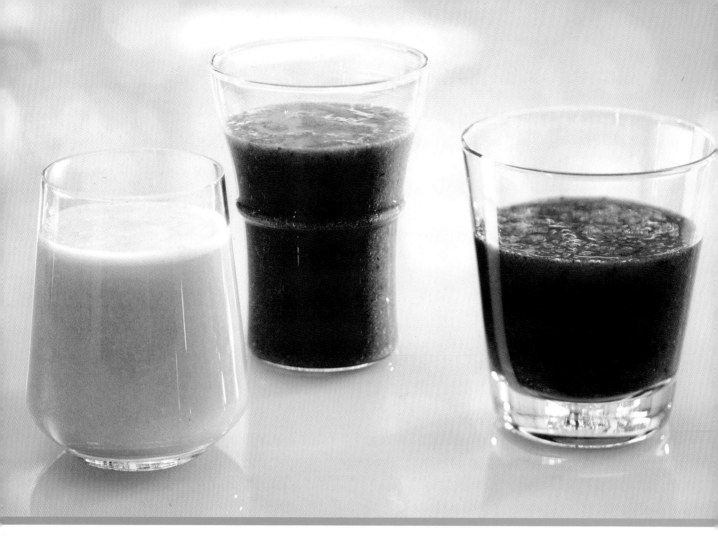

ALL JUICES HAVE A PREPARATION TIME OF **5 MINUTES** & SERVE **1**

ORANGE AND GINGER

3 medium oranges (720g)

2cm piece fresh ginger (10g), grated

1 Juice oranges on citrus squeezer; pour into glass.
2 Stir in ginger.

PER SERVING
0.6g TOTAL FAT
(0g SATURATED FAT)
40.9g CARBOHYDRATE
807kJ (193 CAL)
5.2g PROTEIN
10.5g FIBRE

RASPBERRY AND PEACH

1 large peach (220g), chopped coarsely

¼ cup (35g) raspberries

½ cup (125ml) water

1 Blend or process peach and raspberry until smooth; pour into glass.
2 Stir in the water.

PER SERVING
0.3g TOTAL FAT
(0g SATURATED FAT)
14.1g CARBOHYDRATE
301kJ (72 CAL)
2.1g PROTEIN
4.5g FIBRE

MIXED BERRY

3 strawberries (60g)

¼ cup (40g) blueberries

¼ cup (35g) raspberries

⅓ cup (80ml) water

1 Blend or process ingredients until smooth; pour into glass.
tip For something refreshing, freeze the juice until almost set then scrape with a fork for a granita-like snack.

PER SERVING
0.2g TOTAL FAT
(0g SATURATED FAT)
8.2g CARBOHYDRATE
184kJ (44 CAL)
1.7g PROTEIN
3.9g FIBRE

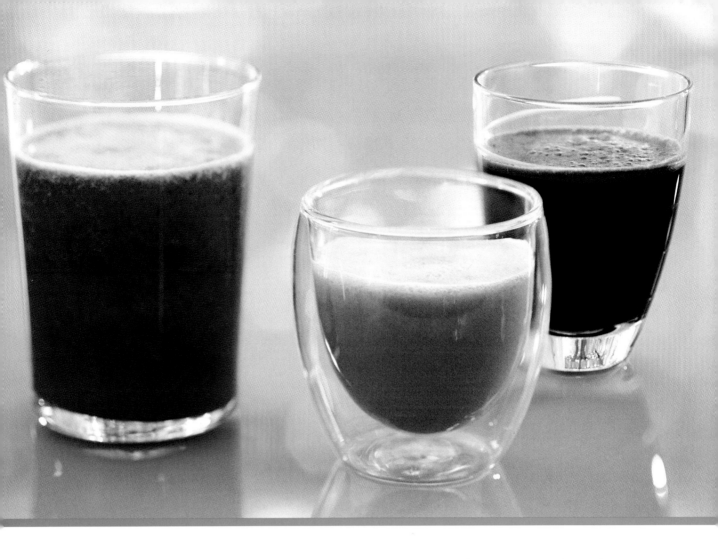

WATERMELON AND MINT

450g watermelon

4 fresh mint leaves

1 Blend or process ingredients until smooth; pour into glass.

PER SERVING
0.6g TOTAL FAT
(0g SATURATED FAT)
14.5g CARBOHYDRATE
280kJ (67 CAL)
0.9g PROTEIN
1.9g FIBRE

PINEAPPLE, ORANGE AND STRAWBERRY

1 small orange (180g), peeled, quartered

150g pineapple, chopped coarsely

2 strawberries (40g)

¼ cup (60ml) water

1 Push orange, pineapple and strawberries through juice extractor into glass; stir in the water.

PER SERVING
0.3g TOTAL FAT
(0g SATURATED FAT)
23.2g CARBOHYDRATE
468kJ (112 CAL)
3.5g PROTEIN
6.6g FIBRE

BEETROOT, CARROT AND SPINACH

1 small beetroot (100g), cut into wedges

1 small carrot (70g), chopped coarsely

20g baby spinach leaves

½ cup (125ml) water

1 Push beetroot, carrot and spinach through juice extractor into glass.
2 Stir in the water.

PER SERVING
0.2g TOTAL FAT
(0g SATURATED FAT)
11.2g CARBOHYDRATE
238kJ (57 CAL)
2.7g PROTEIN
5.3g FIBRE

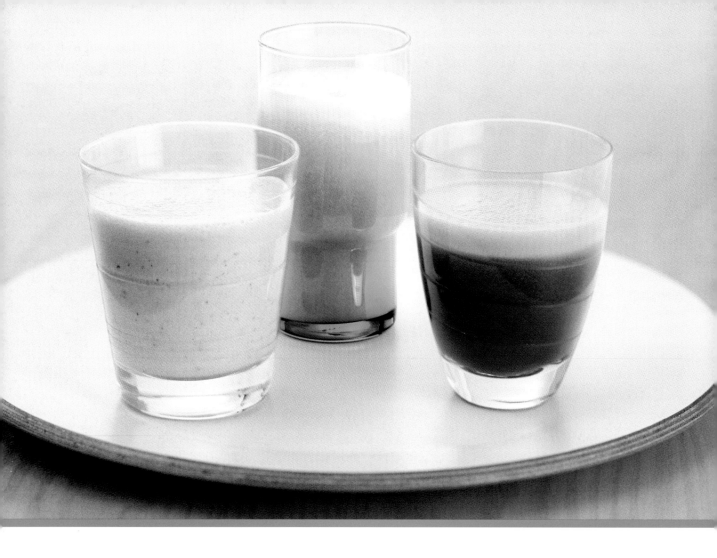

STRAWBERRY, HONEY AND SOY SMOOTHIE

6 strawberries (120g)

½ cup (125ml) soy milk

1 teaspoon honey

1 Blend or process ingredients until smooth; pour into glass.

PER SERVING
3.6g TOTAL FAT
(0.4g SATURATED FAT)
14.4g CARBOHYDRATE
472kJ (113 CAL)
6.2g PROTEIN
3.2g FIBRE

APPLE AND PEAR

We used a green apple in this recipe, but you can use the colour of your choice.

1 medium apple (150g), cut into wedges

1 medium pear (230g), cut into wedges

1 Push ingredients through juice extractor into glass; stir to combine.

PER SERVING
0.4g TOTAL FAT
(0g SATURATED FAT)
51.3g CARBOHYDRATE
853kJ (204 CAL)
1.1g PROTEIN
9g FIBRE

SILVERBEET, APPLE AND CELERY

We used a green apple in this recipe, but you can use the colour of your choice.

1 trimmed silverbeet leaf (80g), chopped coarsely

1 large apple (200g), cut into wedges

1 trimmed celery stalk (100g), chopped coarsely

1 Push ingredients through juice extractor into glass; stir to combine.

PER SERVING
0.5g TOTAL FAT
(0g SATURATED FAT)
24.6g CARBOHYDRATE
460kJ (110 CAL)
2.4g PROTEIN
7.8g FIBRE

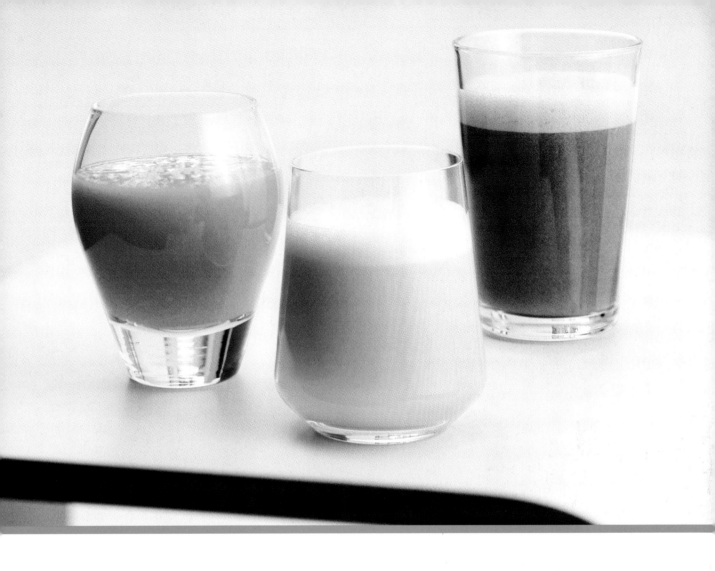

MANGO AND GRAPEFRUIT

1 small grapefruit (350g)

1 small mango (300g), chopped coarsely

¼ cup (60ml) water

1 Juice grapefruit on citrus squeezer; pour into glass.
2 Blend or process mango and the water until smooth. Transfer to same glass; stir to combine.

PER SERVING
0.9g TOTAL FAT
(0g SATURATED FAT)
37.8g CARBOHYDRATE
757kJ (181 CAL)
4.2g PROTEIN
4.6g FIBRE

APPLE AND CELERY

We used green apples in this recipe, but you can use the colour of your choice.

2 small apples (260g), cut into wedges

1 trimmed celery stalk (100g), chopped coarsely

1 Push ingredients through juice extractor into glass; stir to combine.

PER SERVING
0.4g TOTAL FAT
(0g SATURATED FAT)
34.7g CARBOHYDRATE
598kJ (143 CAL)
1.4g PROTEIN
7g FIBRE

PEAR AND GRAPE

1 medium pear (230g), cut into wedges

175g seedless red grapes

1 Push ingredients through juice extractor into glass; stir to combine.

PER SERVING
0.4g TOTAL FAT
(0g SATURATED FAT)
55.6g CARBOHYDRATE
953kJ (228 CAL)
2.8g PROTEIN
7.3g FIBRE

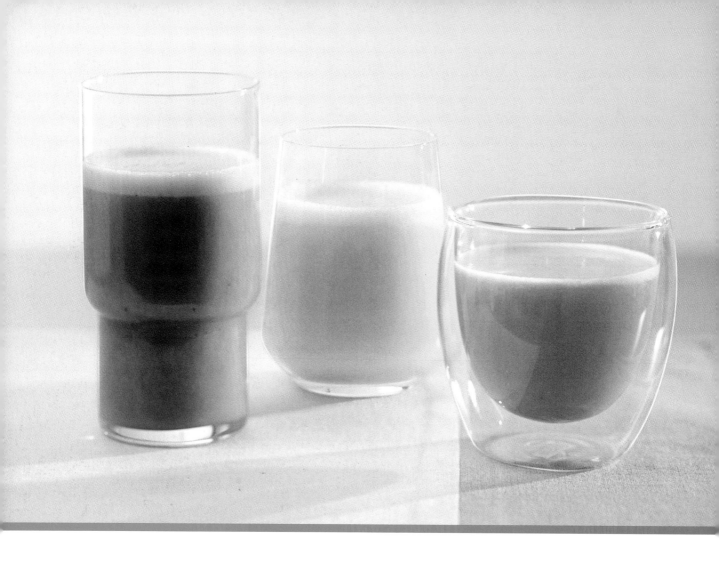

ALL JUICES HAVE A PREPARATION TIME OF **5 MINUTES** & SERVE **1**

PINEAPPLE, GINGER AND MINT

You need ½ small pineapple for this recipe.

400g pineapple, chopped coarsely

1 cup firmly packed fresh mint leaves

1cm piece fresh ginger (5g)

1 Push ingredients through juice extractor into glass; stir to combine.

PER SERVING
0.8g TOTAL FAT
(0.1g SATURATED FAT)
19.1g CARBOHYDRATE
418kJ (100 CAL)
3.7g PROTEIN
8.1g FIBRE

GINGER, ORANGE AND PINEAPPLE

You need ¼ small pineapple for this recipe.

1 medium orange (240g)

200g pineapple, chopped coarsely

2cm piece fresh ginger (10g)

1 Juice orange on citrus squeezer; pour into glass.
2 Blend or process pineapple and ginger until smooth. Stir into orange juice.

PER SERVING
0.3g TOTAL FAT
(0g SATURATED FAT)
22.2g CARBOHYDRATE
439kJ (105 CAL)
2.8g PROTEIN
5.9g FIBRE

MANDARIN

3 small mandarins (300g)

1 Juice mandarins on citrus squeezer; pour into glass.

PER SERVING
0.4g TOTAL FAT
(0g SATURATED FAT)
17g CARBOHYDRATE
343kJ (82 CAL)
1.9g PROTEIN
4.3g FIBRE

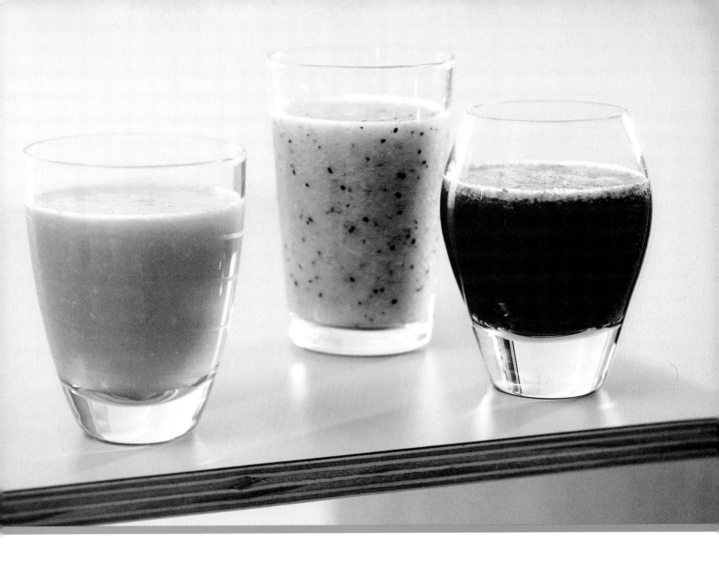

TANGELO
AND GINGER

2 medium tangelos (420g)

**2cm piece fresh ginger
(10g), grated**

1   Juice tangelos on citrus squeezer;
    pour into glass.
2   Stir in ginger.

KIWI FRUIT AND
GREEN GRAPE

**3 medium kiwi fruits (255g),
quartered**

70g seedless green grapes

¼ cup (60ml) water

1   Blend or process ingredients
    until smooth; pour into glass.

GRAPEFRUIT AND
BLOOD ORANGE

2 small blood oranges (360g)

1 small grapefruit (350g)

1   Juice oranges and grapefruit on citrus
    squeezer; pour into glass.

PER SERVING
0.3g TOTAL FAT
(0g SATURATED FAT)
23.7g CARBOHYDRATE
477kJ (114 CAL)
1.9g PROTEIN
6.2g FIBRE

PER SERVING
0.5g TOTAL FAT
(0g SATURATED FAT)
31.8g CARBOHYDRATE
623kJ (149 CAL)
3.5g PROTEIN
7.8g FIBRE

PER SERVING
0.7g TOTAL FAT
(0g SATURATED FAT)
31.2g CARBOHYDRATE
652kJ (156 CAL)
4.6g PROTEIN
6.5g FIBRE

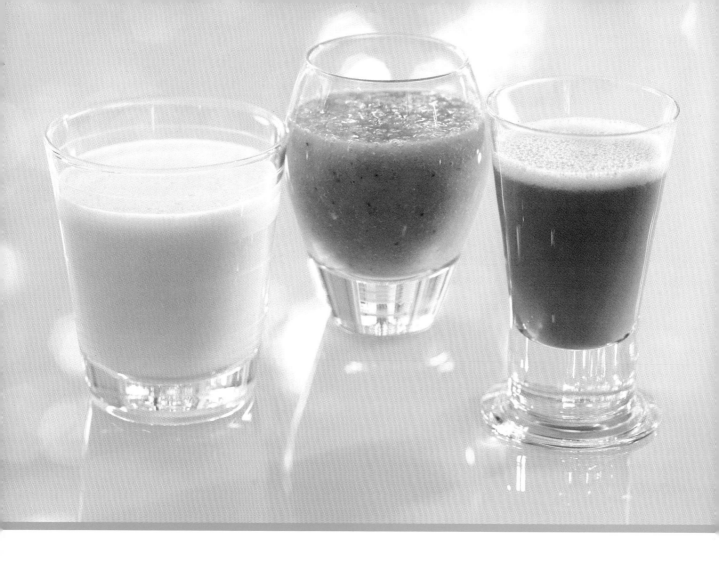

ALL JUICES HAVE A PREPARATION TIME OF **5 MINUTES** & SERVE **1**

PEAR AND GINGER

2 medium pears (460g), cut into wedges

2cm piece fresh ginger (10g)

1 Push ingredients through juice extractor into glass; stir to combine.

PER SERVING
0.5g TOTAL FAT
(0g SATURATED FAT)
52.6g CARBOHYDRATE
882kJ (211 CAL)
1.3g PROTEIN
9.8g FIBRE

ORANGE, MANGO AND STRAWBERRY

2 small oranges (360g)

1 small mango (300g), chopped coarsely

3 strawberries (60g), chopped coarsely

1 Juice oranges on citrus squeezer; pour into glass.
2 Blend or process mango and strawberries until smooth; stir into orange juice.

PER SERVING
0.7g TOTAL FAT
(0g SATURATED FAT)
48.7g CARBOHYDRATE
949kJ (227 CAL)
5.7g PROTEIN
9.6g FIBRE

ORANGE, CARROT AND CELERY

1 large orange (300g), peeled, quartered

1 large carrot (180g), chopped coarsely

1 trimmed celery stalk (100g), chopped coarsely

1 Push orange, carrot and celery through juice extractor into glass; stir to combine.

PER SERVING
0.5g TOTAL FAT
(0g SATURATED FAT)
28.6g CARBOHYDRATE
573kJ (137 CAL)
4.2g PROTEIN
11.3g FIBRE

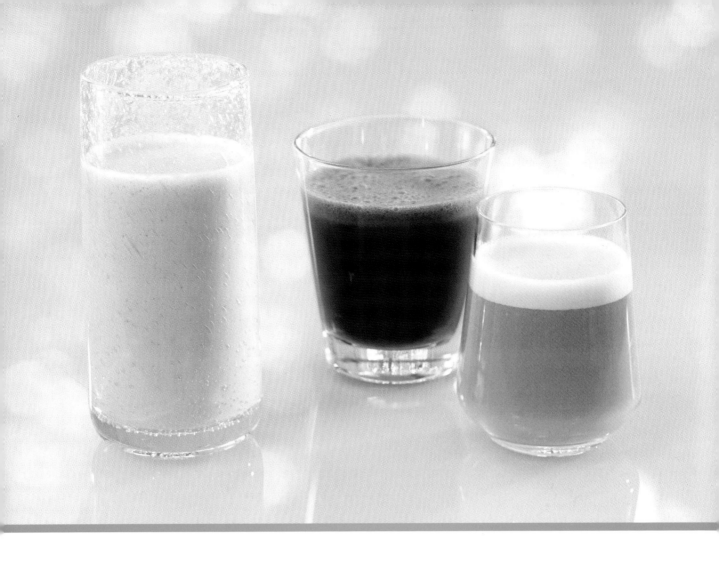

BANANA SOY SMOOTHIE

1 cup (250ml) soy milk

1 small banana (130g), chopped coarsely

1 Blend or process ingredients until smooth; pour into glass.

CARROT, GINGER AND SILVERBEET

2 medium carrots (240g), chopped coarsely

3 trimmed silverbeet leaves (240g), chopped coarsely

2cm piece fresh ginger (10g)

1 Push ingredients through juice extractor into glass; stir to combine.

ORANGE, CARROT AND GINGER

2 medium oranges (480g), peeled, quartered

1 small carrot (70g), chopped coarsely

2cm piece fresh ginger (10g)

1 Push orange, carrot and ginger through juice extractor into glass; stir to combine.

PER SERVING
2.1g TOTAL FAT
(0.2g SATURATED FAT)
8.2g CARBOHYDRATE
255kJ (61 CAL)
8.2g PROTEIN
0.9g FIBRE

PER SERVING
0.7g TOTAL FAT
(0g SATURATED FAT)
14.5g CARBOHYDRATE
364kJ (87 CAL)
5.4g PROTEIN
13.1g FIBRE

PER SERVING
0.4g TOTAL FAT
(0g SATURATED FAT)
30.6g CARBOHYDRATE
606kJ (145 CAL)
4g PROTEIN
8.8g FIBRE

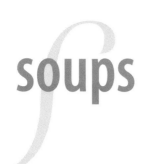

soups

PER 250ML
0.4g TOTAL FAT
(**0G** SATURATED FAT)
15.8g CARBOHYDRATE
343kJ (**82 CAL**)
3.8g PROTEIN
6.5g FIBRE

VEGETABLE STOCK

PREPARATION TIME **30 MINUTES** COOKING TIME **1 HOUR 40 MINUTES** MAKES **2 LITRES**

2 medium brown onions (300g), chopped coarsely

3 medium carrots (360g), chopped coarsely

3 medium parsnips (750g), chopped coarsely

2 medium swedes (450g), chopped coarsely

1 small fennel bulb (200g), chopped coarsely

1 large red capsicum (350g), chopped coarsely

1 trimmed celery stalk (100g), chopped coarsely

2 cloves garlic, chopped coarsely

2 bay leaves

6 black peppercorns

4 litres (16 cups) water

1¼ cups coarsely chopped fresh flat-leaf parsley

1 Combine vegetables, bay leaves, peppercorns and the water in large stock pot or saucepan; bring to a boil. Reduce heat; simmer, uncovered, stirring occasionally, 1 hour. Add parsley; simmer, uncovered, 30 minutes.
2 Strain stock through muslin-lined sieve or colander; discard solids.

tip Stock can be kept, covered, for up to a week in the refrigerator. Stock also suitable to freeze for up to three months.

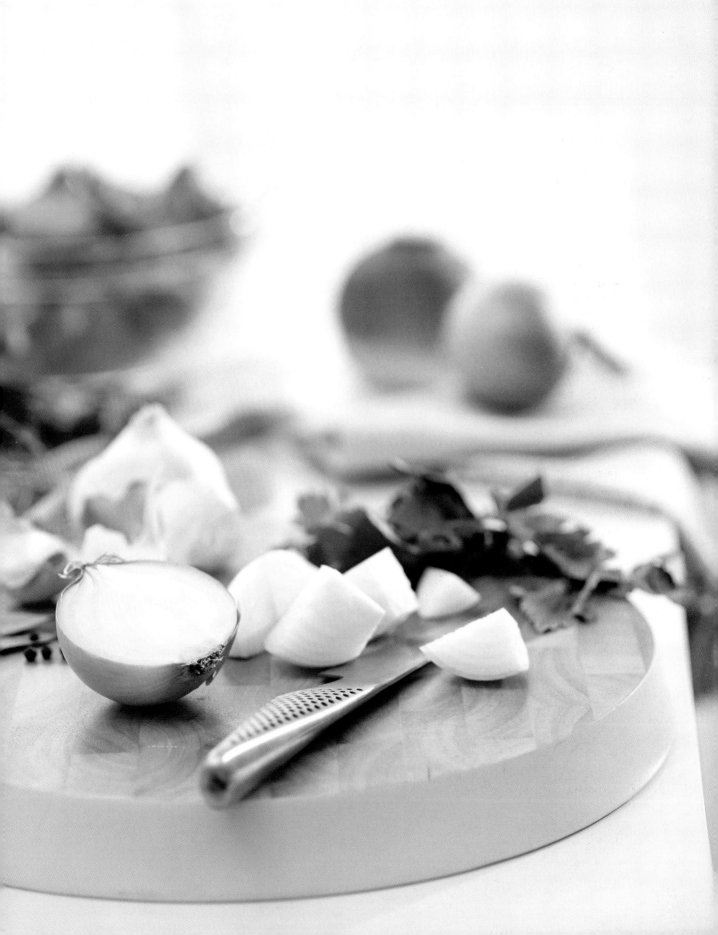

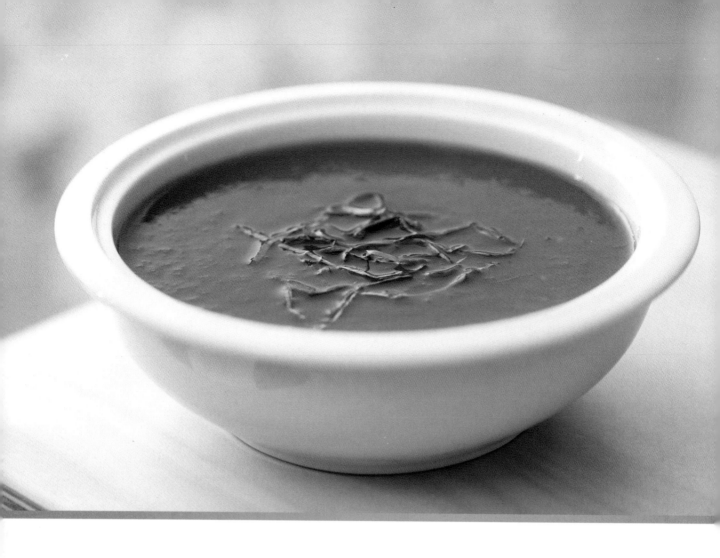

ASIAN BROTH

PREPARATION TIME **15 MINUTES** (PLUS STANDING TIME) COOKING TIME **10 MINUTES** SERVES **1**

PER SERVING
2.6g TOTAL FAT
(0.4g SATURATED FAT)
13.8g CARBOHYDRATE
410kJ (98 CAL)
4.6g PROTEIN
6.6g FIBRE

5 dried shiitake mushrooms (10g)

1½ cups (375ml) vegetable stock (page 50)

2 teaspoons tamari

1cm piece fresh ginger (5g), grated

½ teaspoon peanut oil

½ small carrot (35g), sliced thinly

30g snow peas, trimmed, chopped coarsely

1 green onion, sliced thinly

½ cup (40g) finely shredded chinese cabbage

30g canned bamboo shoots, cut into matchsticks

1 Place mushrooms in small heatproof bowl, cover with boiling water, stand 20 minutes; drain. Discard stems; halve caps.
2 Combine stock, tamari, ginger and oil in medium saucepan; bring to a boil. Add mushroom and carrot, reduce heat; simmer, covered, until carrot is just tender. Add peas, onion, cabbage and bamboo shoots; simmer, uncovered, 2 minutes.

ROASTED TOMATO AND CAPSICUM SOUP

PREPARATION TIME **10 MINUTES** COOKING TIME **35 MINUTES** SERVES **1**

4 large tomatoes (880g), chopped coarsely

1 large red capsicum (350g), chopped coarsely

1 small brown onion (80g), chopped coarsely

2 cloves garlic, sliced thinly

1 tablespoon finely shredded fresh basil

PER SERVING
1.6g TOTAL FAT
(**0g** SATURATED FAT)
33.1g CARBOHYDRATE
895kJ (214 CAL)
14.9g PROTEIN
15.4g FIBRE

1 Preheat oven to moderate (180°C/160°C fan-forced).
2 Combine tomato, capsicum, onion and garlic in small baking dish; roast, covered, about 30 minutes or until vegetables soften.
3 Push vegetables through mouli or fine sieve into small saucepan; discard solids.
4 Reheat soup; serve soup topped with basil.

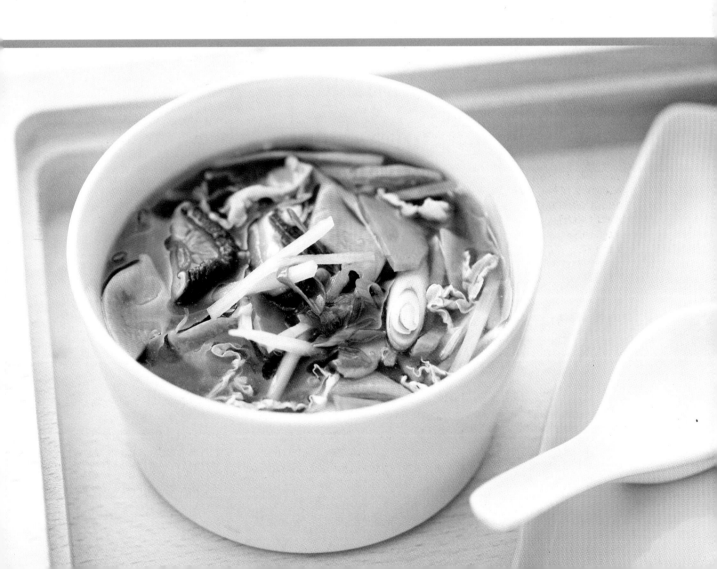

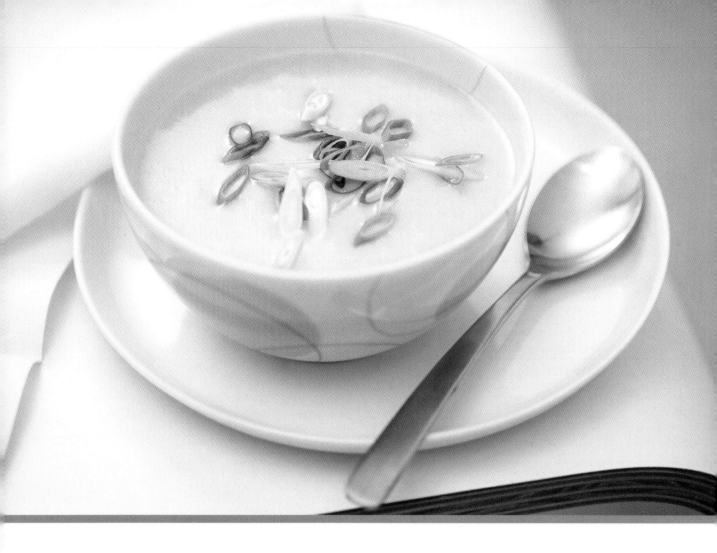

VEGETABLE SOUP

PREPARATION TIME **10 MINUTES** COOKING TIME **20 MINUTES** SERVES **1**

PER SERVING
2.7g TOTAL FAT
(0.2g SATURATED FAT)
45g CARBOHYDRATE
1074kJ (257 CAL)
12.6g PROTEIN
15.3g FIBRE

2 cups (500ml) vegetable stock (page 50)

1 trimmed corn cob (250g)

½ cup (50g) coarsely chopped cauliflower

½ small carrot (35g), diced into 1cm pieces

30g snow peas, trimmed, sliced thinly

1 green onion, sliced thinly

1 Bring stock to a boil in small saucepan. Cut kernels from corn cob, add to pan with cauliflower and carrot; return to a boil. Reduce heat; simmer, covered, about 10 minutes or until cauliflower is just tender.

2 Stir in snow peas and onion; simmer, uncovered, 2 minutes.

LEEK AND POTATO SOUP

PREPARATION TIME **10 MINUTES** COOKING TIME **25 MINUTES** SERVES **1**

1 teaspoon olive oil

1 clove garlic, crushed

½ teaspoon fresh thyme leaves

1 small leek (200g), sliced thinly

1 medium potato (200g), chopped coarsely

2 cups (500ml) vegetable stock (page 50)

½ green onion, sliced thinly

PER SERVING
5.5g TOTAL FAT
(0.7g SATURATED FAT)
38.5g CARBOHYDRATE
1016kJ (243 CAL)
9.3g PROTEIN
11.1g FIBRE

1 Heat oil in small saucepan; cook garlic, thyme and leek, stirring, about 3 minutes or until leek softens. Add potato and stock; bring to a boil. Reduce heat; simmer, covered, about 15 minutes or until potato is tender.

2 Blend or process leek mixture until smooth.

3 Reheat soup; serve soup topped with onion.

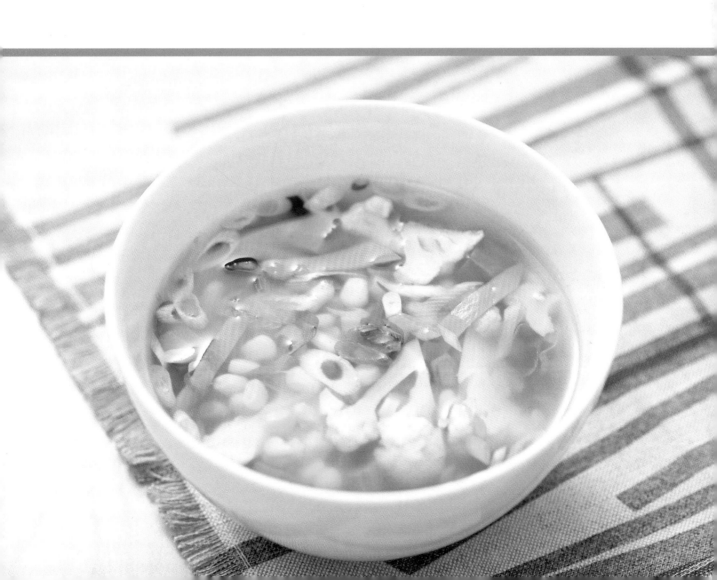

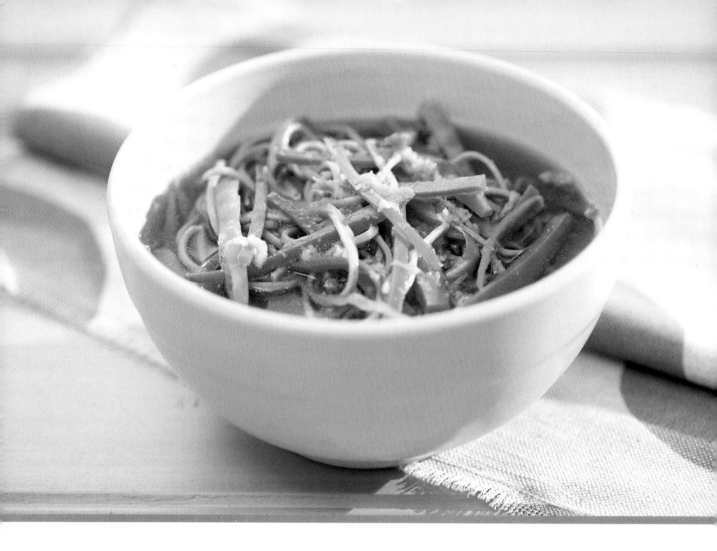

PUMPKIN AND KUMARA SOUP

PREPARATION TIME **15 MINUTES** COOKING TIME **25 MINUTES** SERVES **1**

PER SERVING
6g TOTAL FAT
(**1.3g** SATURATED FAT)
60.1g CARBOHYDRATE
1438kJ (344 CAL)
12.2g PROTEIN
12.2g FIBRE

1 teaspoon olive oil

1 small brown onion (80g), chopped coarsely

1 clove garlic, crushed

200g pumpkin, chopped coarsely

1 small kumara (250g), chopped coarsely

2 cups (500ml) vegetable stock (page 50)

¼ teaspoon finely grated orange rind

1 tablespoon fresh orange juice

1 tablespoon finely chopped fresh chives

1 Heat oil in medium saucepan; cook onion and garlic, stirring, until onion softens.
2 Add pumpkin, kumara and stock; bring to a boil. Reduce heat; simmer, covered, about 15 minutes or until pumpkin and kumara are tender. Cool 10 minutes.
3 Blend or process pumpkin mixture until smooth.
4 Return soup mixture to same pan with rind and juice; stir over heat, without boiling, until heated through.
5 Serve soup topped with chives.

VEGETABLE AND SOBA SOUP

PREPARATION TIME **15 MINUTES** COOKING TIME **15 MINUTES** SERVES **1**

Soba is a Japanese noodle, similar in appearance to spaghetti, made from buckwheat.

2 cups (500ml) vegetable stock (page 50)

1 teaspoon tamari

5cm piece fresh ginger (25g), grated

2 cloves garlic, crushed

1 small carrot (70g), cut into matchsticks

50g snow peas, trimmed, sliced thinly lengthways

50g soba

PER SERVING
1.2g TOTAL FAT
(**0.2g** SATURATED FAT)
51.8g CARBOHYDRATE
1108kJ (**265 CAL**)
10.9g PROTEIN
10.5g FIBRE

1 Combine stock, tamari, ginger and garlic in small saucepan; bring to a boil. Reduce heat; simmer, covered, 5 minutes. Add carrot and snow peas; simmer, uncovered, about 3 minutes or until carrot is tender.
2 Meanwhile, cook noodles in small saucepan of boiling water, uncovered, until just tender; drain.
3 Place noodles in serving bowl; ladle soup over noodles.

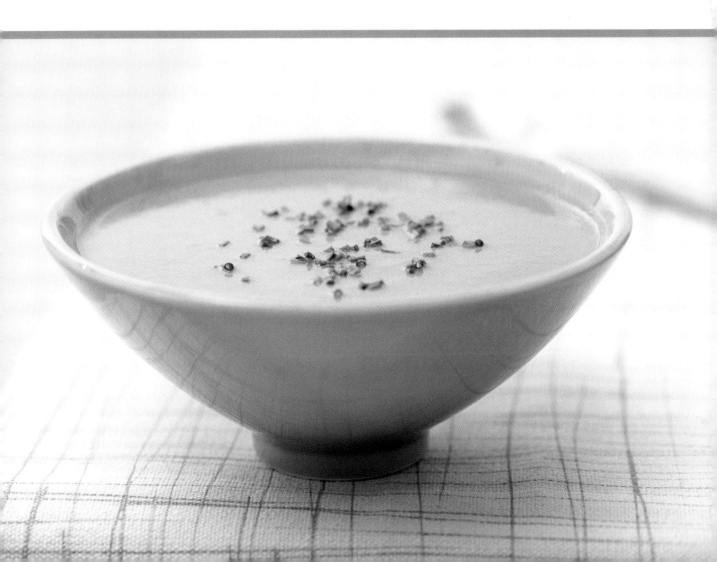

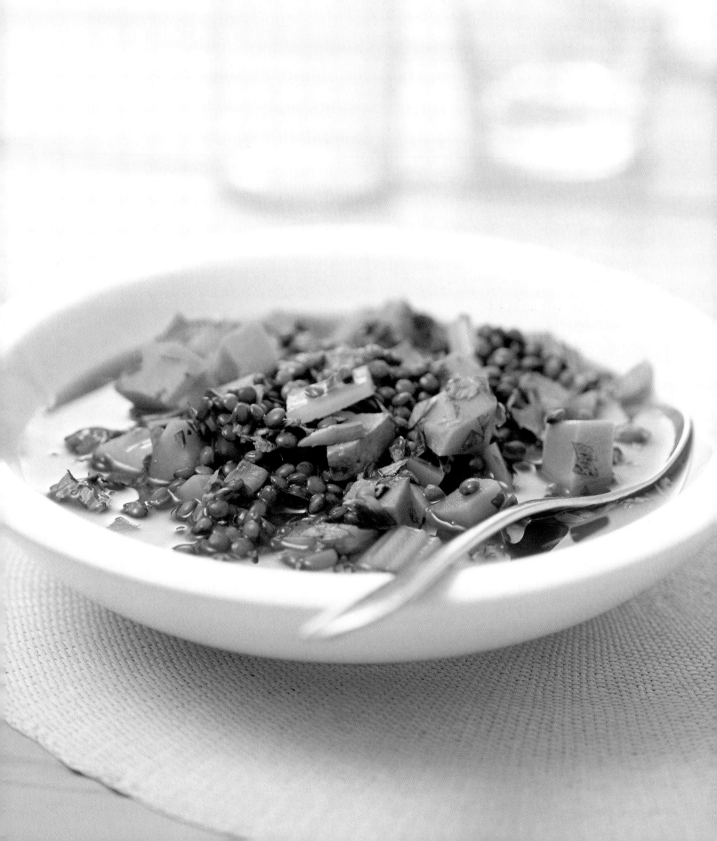

PER SERVING
1.7g TOTAL FAT
(0.2g SATURATED FAT)
37.5g CARBOHYDRATE
978kJ (234 CAL)
18g PROTEIN
17.7g FIBRE

LENTIL AND VEGETABLE SOUP

PREPARATION TIME **10 MINUTES** COOKING TIME **45 MINUTES** SERVES **1**

French green lentils have a sensational nutty, earthy flavour and
stand up well to being boiled without becoming muddy. They are
available at specialist food shops and better delicatessens.
You need the leaves from the celery stalk for this recipe.

2 cups (500ml) vegetable stock (page 50)

¼ cup (50g) french green lentils

1 clove garlic, crushed

½ untrimmed celery stalk (75g)

1 medium carrot (120g), chopped coarsely

50g mushrooms, chopped coarsely

2 tablespoons coarsely chopped fresh flat-leaf parsley

1 Combine stock, lentils, garlic and celery leaves in small saucepan; bring to a boil. Reduce
   heat; simmer, covered, about 20 minutes or until lentils just soften. Discard celery leaves.
2 Add coarsely chopped celery stalk, carrot and mushroom; bring to a boil. Reduce heat;
   simmer, covered, about 15 minutes or until vegetables are tender. Stir in parsley.

vegetable dishes

PER SERVING
19.6g TOTAL FAT
(**3.1g** SATURATED FAT)
6.1g CARBOHYDRATE
1221kJ (292 CAL)
23g PROTEIN
12.8g FIBRE

STIR-FRIED ASIAN GREENS WITH TOFU

PREPARATION TIME **10 MINUTES** COOKING TIME **10 MINUTES** SERVES **1**

2 teaspoons peanut oil

2cm piece fresh ginger (10g), cut into slivers

1 clove garlic, crushed

100g gai larn, chopped coarsely

100g broccolini, chopped coarsely

150g baby bok choy, chopped coarsely

100g firm tofu, chopped coarsely

1 tablespoon water

2 teaspoons tamari

2 teaspoons coarsely chopped toasted peanuts

1 Heat oil in wok; stir-fry ginger and garlic until fragrant. Add vegetables, tofu, the water and tamari; stir-fry until greens are just tender.
2 Serve stir-fry sprinkled with nuts.

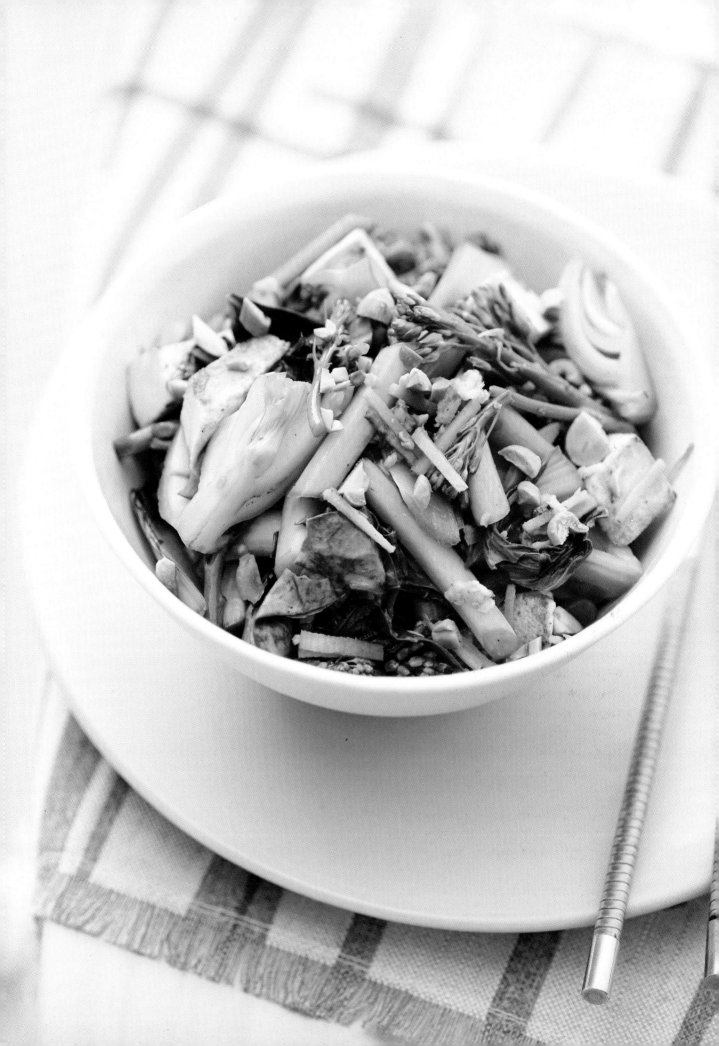

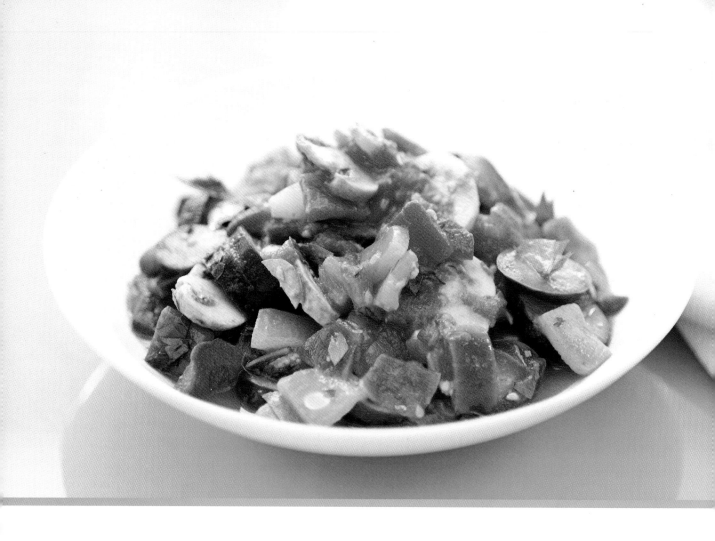

ROASTED CHERRY TOMATOES, BROCCOLINI AND PEPITAS

PREPARATION TIME **10 MINUTES** COOKING TIME **20 MINUTES** SERVES **1**

PER SERVING
16.7g TOTAL FAT
(0.7g SATURATED FAT)
10.3g CARBOHYDRATE
1379kJ (330 CAL)
14.2g PROTEIN
17.9g FIBRE

1 teaspoon olive oil

1 small red onion (100g), sliced thinly

2 cloves garlic, crushed

125g cherry tomatoes, halved

1 tablespoon cider vinegar

250g broccolini

2 tablespoons toasted pepitas

1 Preheat oven to moderately hot (200°C/180°C fan-forced).
2 Combine oil and onion in small baking dish; roast, uncovered, 10 minutes. Add garlic, tomato and vinegar; roast, uncovered, about 10 minutes or until tomato softens.
3 Meanwhile, boil, steam or microwave broccolini until tender; drain.
4 Serve broccollini topped with tomato mixture and seeds.

RATATOUILLE

PREPARATION TIME **20 MINUTES** COOKING TIME **25 MINUTES** SERVES **1**

1 small red capsicum (150g)

1 small yellow capsicum (150g)

1 teaspoon olive oil

1 clove garlic, crushed

½ small red onion (50g), chopped coarsely

1 baby eggplant (60g), sliced thickly

1 small zucchini (90g), sliced thickly

2 large tomatoes (440g), peeled, chopped coarsely

100g mushrooms, sliced thickly

1 tablespoon fresh lemon juice

1 tablespoon coarsely chopped fresh flat-leaf parsley

PER SERVING
6.2g TOTAL FAT
(0.7g SATURATED FAT)
23.9g CARBOHYDRATE
895kJ (214 CAL)
14.3g PROTEIN
13.9g FIBRE

1 Quarter capsicums; discard seeds and membranes. Roast under grill or in very hot oven, skin-side up, until skin blisters and blackens. Cover capsicum pieces with plastic or paper for 5 minutes; peel away skin then chop capsicum coarsely.

2 Meanwhile, heat oil in medium saucepan; cook garlic, onion, eggplant, zucchini, tomato and mushroom, covered, over medium heat, stirring occasionally, 10 minutes. Stir in capsicum; cook, uncovered, until heated through. Stir in juice and parsley.

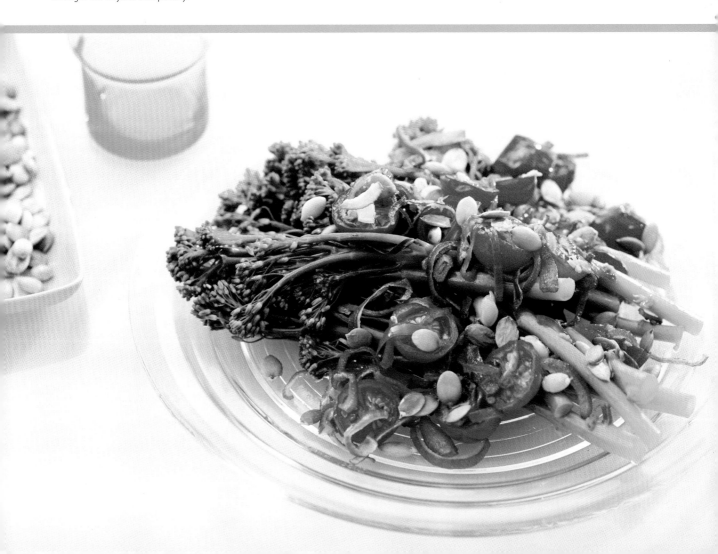

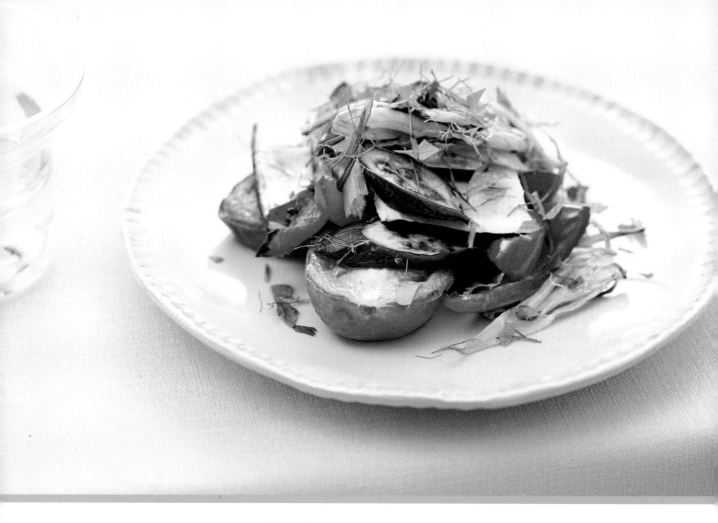

BLACK-EYED BEANS WITH KUMARA, SHALLOTS AND GARLIC

PREPARATION TIME **20 MINUTES** (PLUS STANDING TIME) COOKING TIME **35 MINUTES** SERVES **1**

PER SERVING
6.1g TOTAL FAT
(0.8g SATURATED FAT)
39.1g CARBOHYDRATE
1078kJ (258 CAL)
10.3g PROTEIN
12.1g FIBRE

⅓ cup (65g) dried black-eyed beans

1 teaspoon olive oil

5 shallots (125g)

5 cloves garlic, unpeeled

1 small kumara (250g), chopped coarsely

2 tablespoons fresh lemon juice

1 small radicchio, shredded finely

1 tablespoon finely chopped fresh flat-leaf parsley

1 Place beans in small bowl, cover with water; stand overnight, drain. Rinse under cold water; drain.
2 Preheat oven to moderately hot (200°C/180°C fan-forced).
3 Combine oil, shallots, garlic and kumara on oven tray. Roast, uncovered, about 20 minutes or until garlic softens. Remove garlic from tray. Return remaining vegetables to oven; roast, uncovered, about 15 minutes or until vegetables are browned lightly.
4 Meanwhile, place beans in small saucepan of boiling water; bring to a boil. Reduce heat; simmer, covered, about 25 minutes or until beans are tender. Drain.
5 Using fingers, squeeze garlic from skins into medium bowl; stir in juice.
6 Add beans, vegetables, radicchio and parsley; toss gently to combine.

ROASTED VEGETABLE STACK

PREPARATION TIME **10 MINUTES** COOKING TIME **20 MINUTES** SERVES **1**

1 baby fennel bulb (130g)

1 medium egg tomato (75g), halved lengthways

½ small red capsicum (75g), sliced thickly

½ medium zucchini (60g), sliced thickly lengthways

1 baby eggplant (60g), sliced thickly

cooking-oil spray

1 tablespoon finely chopped fresh flat-leaf parsley

1 tablespoon fresh lemon juice

1 teaspoon olive oil

PER SERVING

7.2g TOTAL FAT

(0.8g SATURATED FAT)

9.7g CARBOHYDRATE

514kJ (123 CAL)

4.1g PROTEIN

6.5g FIBRE

1 Preheat oven to moderately hot (200°C/180°C fan-forced).

2 Reserve fennel tips from fennel; slice fennel thinly.

3 Place vegetables on lightly oiled oven tray; spray with oil. Roast, uncovered, about 20 minutes or until vegetables soften. Stir in half of the parsley.

4 Stack vegetables on serving plate; drizzle with combined juice and oil, sprinkle with remaining parsley and coarsely chopped reserved fennel tips.

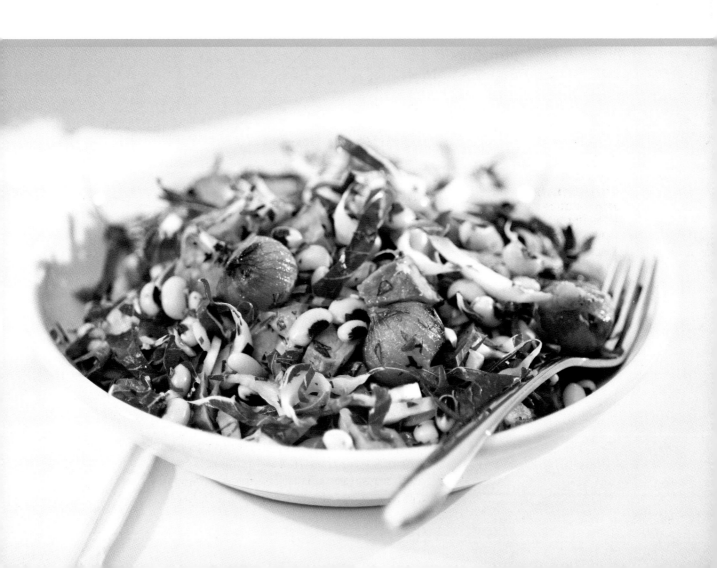

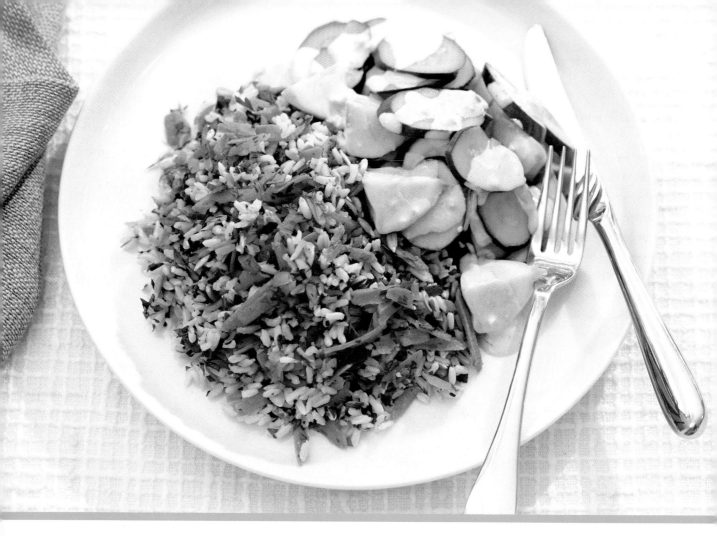

DHAL WITH VEGETABLES

PREPARATION TIME **10 MINUTES** COOKING TIME **35 MINUTES** SERVES **1**

PER SERVING
10g TOTAL FAT
(0.8g SATURATED FAT)
54.8g CARBOHYDRATE
1764kJ (422 CAL)
27.3g PROTEIN
14.5g FIBRE

1 teaspoon vegetable oil

2cm piece fresh ginger (10g), grated

4cm piece fresh turmeric (20g), grated

1 clove garlic, crushed

½ cup (100g) yellow split peas

1 small carrot (70g), chopped coarsely

2 cups (500ml) water

1 small zucchini (90g), chopped coarsely

GINGER YOGURT

1 tablespoon finely chopped fresh coriander

1cm piece fresh ginger (5g), grated

1 tablespoon fresh lime juice

2 tablespoons sheep milk yogurt

1 Heat oil in medium saucepan; cook ginger, turmeric and garlic, stirring, until fragrant.
Add peas, carrot and the water; bring to a boil. Reduce heat; simmer, covered, about
25 minutes or until peas are almost tender. Add zucchini; cook, covered, about 5 minutes
or until zucchini is just tender.

2 Meanwhile, combine ingredients for ginger yogurt in small bowl.

3 Serve dhal with ginger yogurt.

BROWN RICE WITH VEGETABLES AND TAHINI DRESSING

PREPARATION TIME **15 MINUTES** COOKING TIME **20 MINUTES** SERVES **1**

PER SERVING
24.4g TOTAL FAT
(**2.7g** SATURATED FAT)
46.6g CARBOHYDRATE
1965kJ (**470 CAL**)
16g PROTEIN
12.6g FIBRE

¼ cup (50g) brown long-grain rice

1 small zucchini (90g), sliced thinly

2 medium yellow patty-pan squash (60g), quartered

1 small carrot (70g), grated coarsely

¼ cup finely chopped fresh flat-leaf parsley

1 tablespoon sunflower seeds

TAHINI DRESSING

1 tablespoon tahini

2 teaspoons fresh lemon juice

1 tablespoon water

1 clove garlic, crushed

1 Cook rice in small saucepan of boiling water, uncovered, until rice is tender; drain.
2 Meanwhile, boil, steam or microwave zucchini and squash, separately, until tender; drain.
3 Combine rice in small bowl with carrot, parsley and seeds.
4 Place ingredients for tahini dressing in screw-top jar; shake well.
5 Serve rice and vegetables drizzled with dressing.

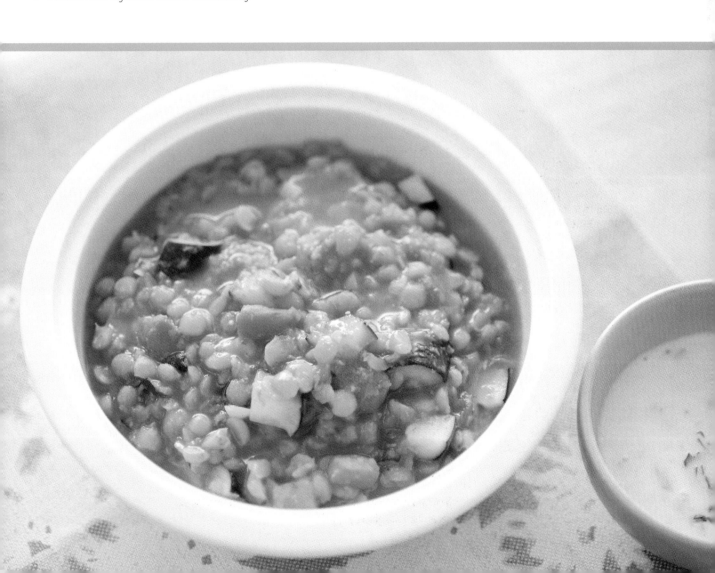

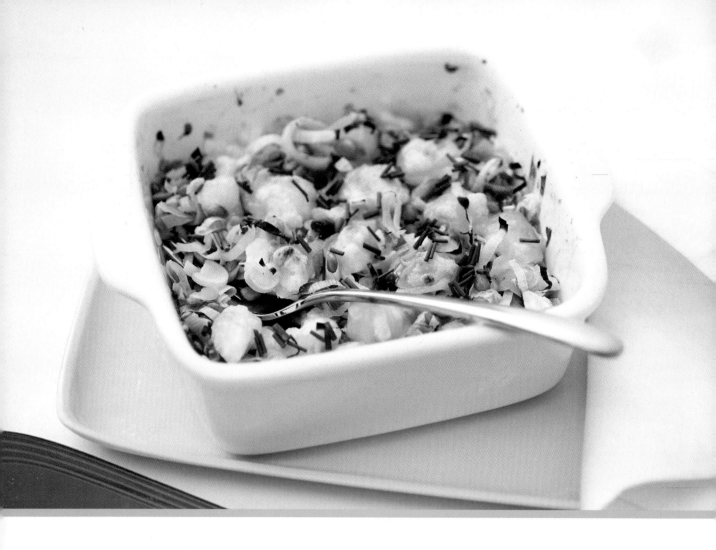

BAKED POTATO WITH GUACAMOLE

PREPARATION TIME **15 MINUTES** COOKING TIME **1 HOUR** SERVES **1**

1 medium potato (200g)

1 small avocado (200g)

½ small red onion (50g), chopped finely

1 small tomato (90g), seeded, chopped finely

1 tablespoon finely chopped fresh coriander

1 tablespoon fresh lime juice

50g mesclun

1 Preheat oven to moderately hot (200°C/180°C fan-forced).
2 Pierce potato skin in several places with fork, wrap potato in foil; place on oven tray.
   Bake about 1 hour or until tender.
3 Mash avocado coarsely in small bowl; stir in onion, tomato, coriander and juice.
4 Cut a deep cross in potato; serve potato topped with guacamole accompanied with mesclun.

LEEK, GOAT CHEESE AND BROWN LENTIL BAKE

PREPARATION TIME **15 MINUTES** COOKING TIME **1 HOUR** SERVES **1**

⅓ cup (65g) brown lentils

1 bay leaf

1 medium leek (350g), sliced thinly

2 tablespoons fresh lemon juice

2 cloves garlic, crushed

¼ cup (60ml) vegetable stock (page 50)

40g goat cheese, crumbled

1 tablespoon coarsely chopped fresh chives

PER SERVING
7.6g TOTAL FAT
(4.2g SATURATED FAT)
18.1g CARBOHYDRATE
819kJ **(196 CAL)**
13.2g PROTEIN
9.8g FIBRE

1 Preheat oven to moderate (180°C/160°C fan-forced).
2 Combine lentils and bay leaf in small saucepan, cover with water; bring to a boil. Reduce heat; simmer, covered, about 10 minutes or until lentils are almost tender. Drain; discard bay leaf.
3 Combine lentils, leek, juice, garlic and stock in 3-cup (750ml) ovenproof dish. Bake, covered, about 40 minutes or until the leek is tender, stirring halfway through cooking.
4 Preheat grill.
5 Sprinkle lentil mixture with cheese; place under grill about 3 minutes or until cheese browns lightly. Sprinkle with chives.

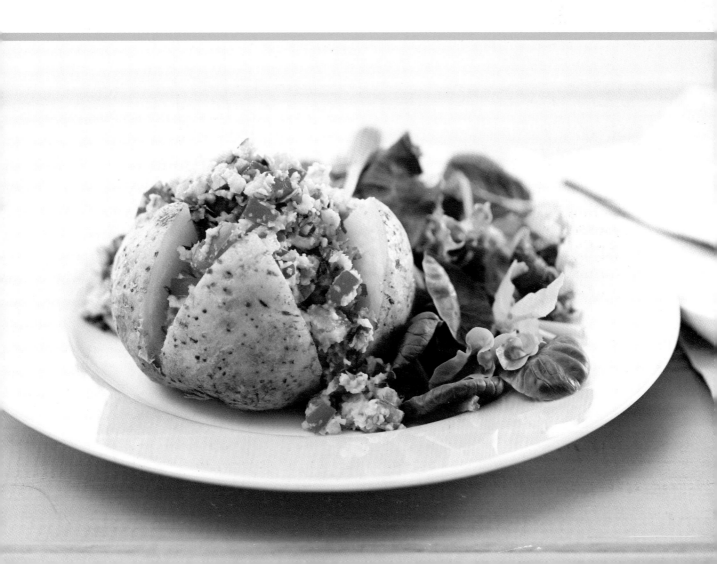

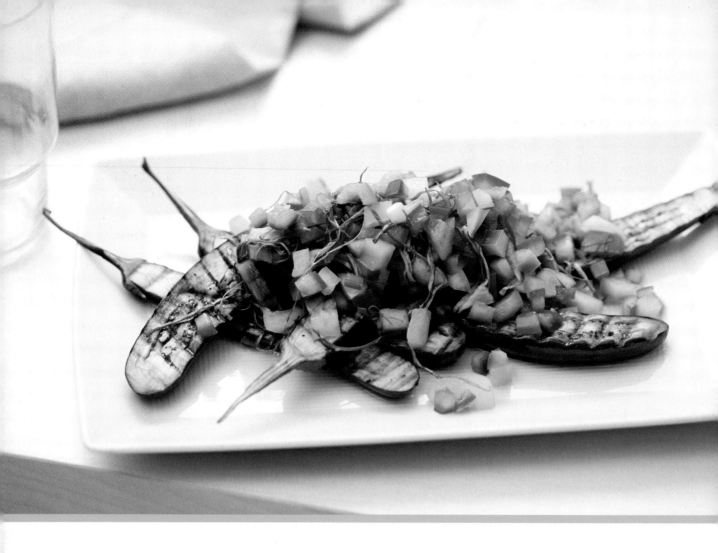

ROASTED ROOT VEGETABLES WITH YOGURT

PREPARATION TIME **15 MINUTES** COOKING TIME **35 MINUTES** SERVES **1**

PER SERVING
12.2g TOTAL FAT
(**2.8g** SATURATED FAT)
51.3g CARBOHYDRATE
1542kJ (**369 CAL**)
13.2g PROTEIN
12.3g FIBRE

1 small parsnip (120g), chopped coarsely

100g celeriac, chopped coarsely

150g pumpkin, chopped coarsely

1 medium potato (200g), chopped coarsely

2 cloves garlic, crushed

1 teaspoon finely chopped fresh rosemary

2 teaspoons olive oil

½ small red capsicum (75g), chopped finely

1 tablespoon coarsely chopped fresh chives

2 tablespoons goat milk yogurt

1 Preheat oven to moderately hot (200°C/180°C fan-forced).
2 Combine parsnip, celeriac, pumpkin, potato, garlic, rosemary and oil on oven tray. Roast, uncovered, about 35 minutes or until vegetables are tender. Add capsicum and chives; toss gently to combine.
3 Serve vegetables topped with yogurt and lemon wedges, if desired.

EGGPLANT WITH SALSA FRESCA

PREPARATION TIME **15 MINUTES** COOKING TIME **15 MINUTES** SERVES **1**

3 baby eggplants (180g), halved lengthways

SALSA FRESCA

½ small green capsicum (75g), chopped finely

½ small yellow capsicum (75g), chopped finely

1 small tomato (90g), seeded, chopped finely

2 tablespoons finely shredded fresh basil

2 tablespoons fresh lemon juice

PER SERVING
0.8g TOTAL FAT
(0g SATURATED FAT)
9.6g CARBOHYDRATE
288kJ (69 CAL)
4.6g PROTEIN
5.9g FIBRE

1 Cook eggplant on heated lightly oiled grill plate (or grill or barbecue) until tender.
2 Combine ingredients for salsa fresca in small bowl.
3 Serve grilled eggplant topped with salsa fresca.

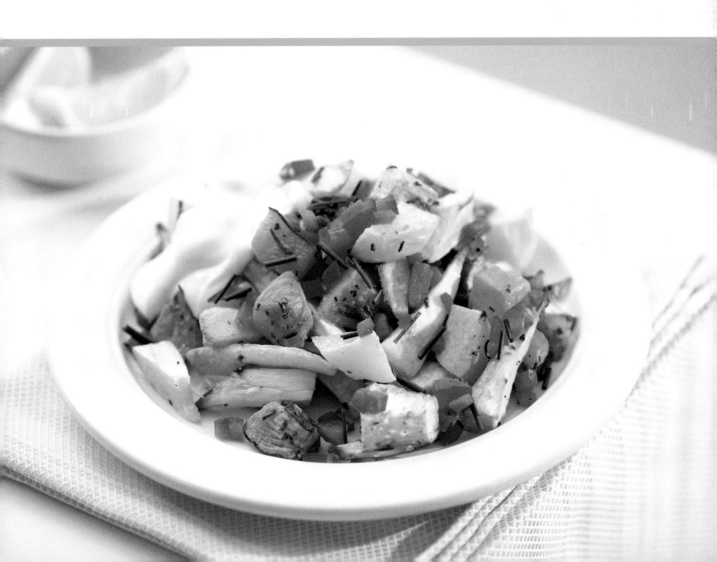

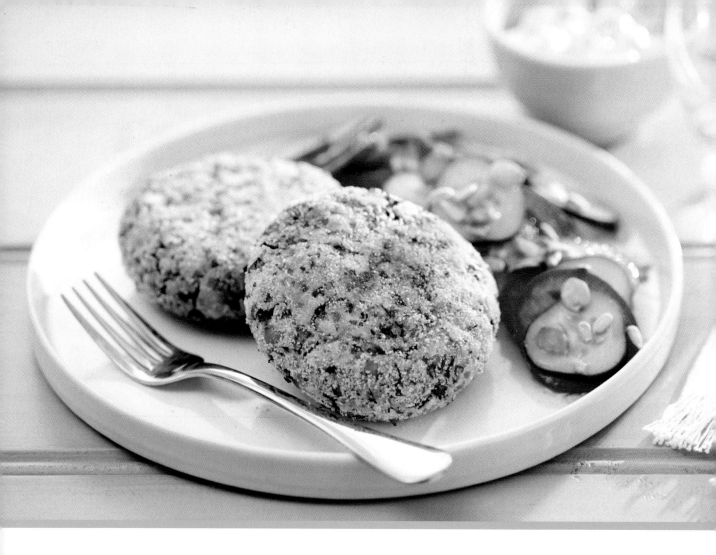

STIR-FRIED ASIAN GREENS WITH MIXED MUSHROOMS

PREPARATION TIME **10 MINUTES** COOKING TIME **5 MINUTES** SERVES **1**

PER SERVING
10.7g TOTAL FAT
(1.3g SATURATED FAT)
7.4g CARBOHYDRATE
757kJ (181 CAL)
13.9g PROTEIN
15.2g FIBRE

2 teaspoons sesame oil

1 clove garlic, crushed

10cm stick (20g) finely chopped fresh lemon grass

2cm piece fresh ginger (10g), grated

150g oyster mushrooms, chopped coarsely

150g button mushrooms, chopped coarsely

150g baby bok choy, chopped coarsely

¼ small chinese cabbage (175g), chopped coarsely

1 Heat oil in wok; stir-fry garlic, lemon grass, ginger and mushrooms until browned
   lightly. Add bok choy and cabbage; stir-fry until greens are just wilted.
2 Serve stir-fry with lime wedges, if desired.

CHICKPEA PATTIES WITH TOMATO AND CUCUMBER SALAD

PREPARATION TIME **20 MINUTES** (PLUS REFRIGERATION TIME) COOKING TIME **40 MINUTES** SERVES **1**

1 medium potato (200g)

300g can chickpeas, rinsed, drained

1 clove garlic, crushed

1 green onion, sliced thinly

⅓ cup coarsely chopped fresh coriander

1 tablespoon polenta

1 lebanese cucumber (130g)

1 small egg tomato (60g), sliced thickly

1 tablespoon fresh lime juice

1 teaspoon pepitas

1 teaspoon sesame seeds

¼ cup (70g) sheep milk yogurt

PER SERVING

21.1g TOTAL FAT

(1.4g SATURATED FAT)

64.6g CARBOHYDRATE

2491kJ (596 CAL)

24.5g PROTEIN

18.5g FIBRE

1 Boil, steam or microwave potato until tender; drain. Mash potato and chickpeas in medium bowl; stir in garlic, onion and coriander. Using hands; shape mixture into two patties. Coat with polenta; refrigerate 1 hour.

2 Cook patties in lightly oiled medium frying pan until browned lightly. Transfer to oven tray; bake in preheated moderate oven (180°C/160°C fan-forced) about 15 minutes or until patties are heated through.

3 Meanwhile, slice half of the cucumber thinly; combine in medium bowl with tomato, juice and seeds. Cut remaining cucumber coarsely; combine in small bowl with yogurt. Serve patties with salad and yogurt.

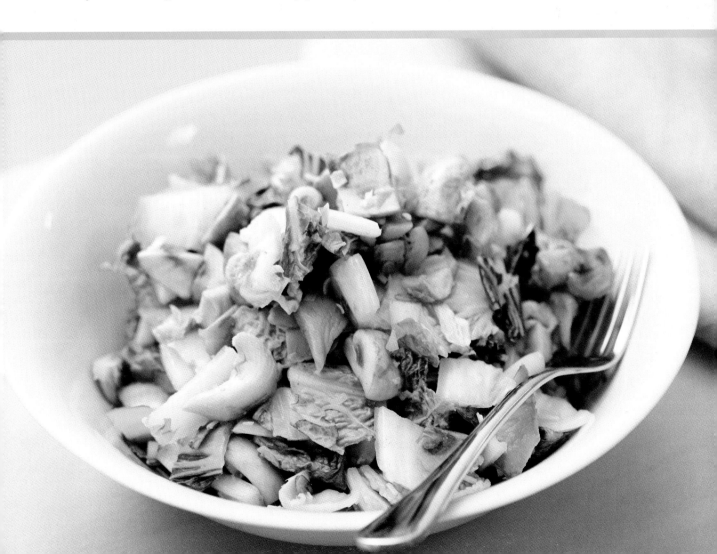

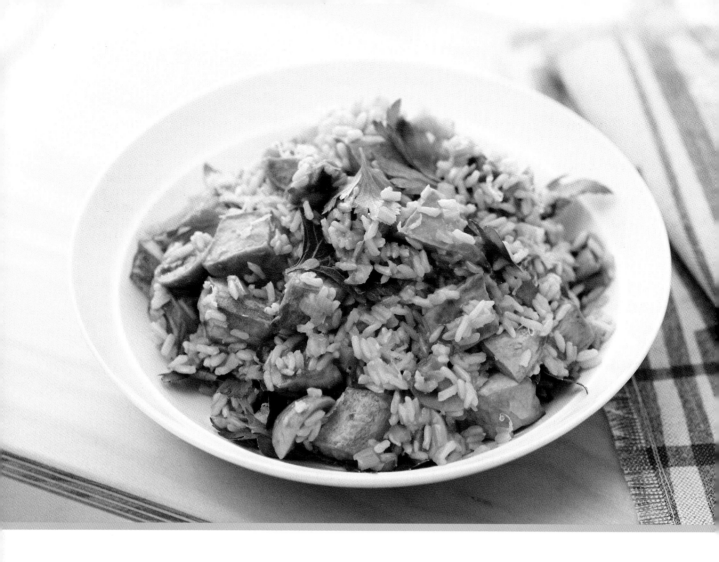

STIR-FRIED TOFU WITH VEGETABLES AND LEMON GRASS

PREPARATION TIME **10 MINUTES** COOKING TIME **5 MINUTES** SERVES **1**

PER SERVING
12.4g TOTAL FAT
(**1.7g** SATURATED FAT)
9.7g CARBOHYDRATE
924kJ (221 CAL)
17.7g PROTEIN
8.2g FIBRE

1 teaspoon sesame oil

100g firm tofu, diced into 1cm pieces

1 small red capsicum (150g), sliced thinly

300g baby bok choy, chopped coarsely

10cm stick (20g) finely chopped fresh lemon grass

1 clove garlic, crushed

¼ cup loosely packed fresh coriander leaves

1 Heat oil in wok; stir-fry tofu, capsicum, bok choy, lemon grass and garlic until vegetables are just tender. Stir in coriander.
2 Serve stir-fry with lemon wedges, if desired.

BROWN RICE PILAF

PREPARATION TIME **15 MINUTES** COOKING TIME **1 HOUR** SERVES **1**

1 small kumara (250g), chopped coarsely

cooking-oil spray

1½ cups (375ml) vegetable stock (page 50)

1 teaspoon olive oil

1 small brown onion (80g), chopped finely

1 clove garlic, crushed

1 trimmed celery stalk (100g), chopped finely

70g mushrooms, chopped coarsely

¾ cup (150g) brown medium-grain rice

1 tablespoon finely grated lemon rind

¼ cup loosely packed fresh flat-leaf parsley leaves

PER SERVING
11.1g TOTAL FAT
(**1.6g** SATURATED FAT)
161.4g CARBOHYDRATE
3515kJ (**841 CAL**)
22.2g PROTEIN
18g FIBRE

1 Preheat oven to moderate (180°C/160°C fan-forced).

2 Place kumara on lightly oiled oven tray; spray with oil. Roast, uncovered, about 25 minutes or until tender.

3 Meanwhile, bring stock to a boil in small saucepan. Reduce heat; simmer, uncovered.

4 Heat oil in medium saucepan; cook onion, garlic and celery, stirring, until onion softens. Add mushroom and rice; cook, stirring, 2 minutes. Add stock, reduce heat; simmer, covered, about 50 minutes or until stock is absorbed and rice is tender. Stir in kumara, rind and parsley.

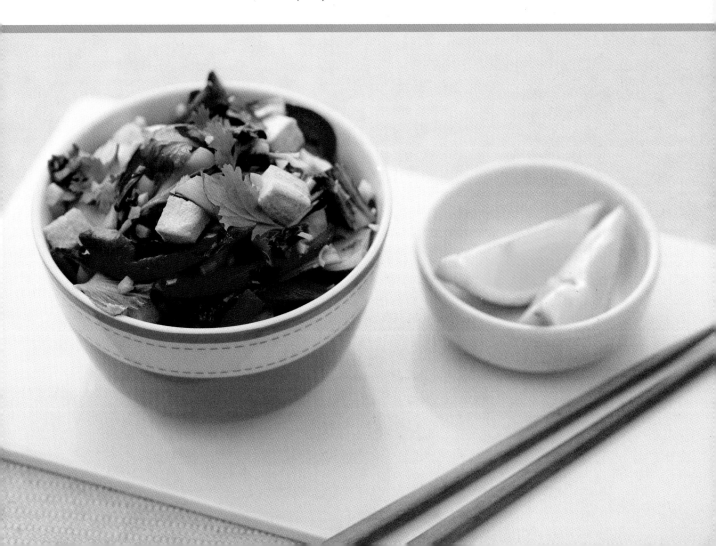

These yummy dips are best served with assorted crudités such as carrot, cucumber and capsicum sticks. All dips are enough to serve 1.

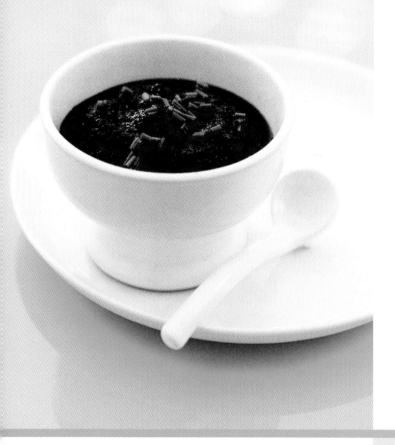

BEETROOT DIP

PREPARATION TIME **5 MINUTES**

225g can beetroot slices, drained
¼ cup (70g) sheep milk yogurt

1 Blend or process beetroot with yogurt.
2 Serve beetroot dip sprinkled with coarsely chopped chives, if desired.

PER SERVING
4.4g TOTAL FAT
(0g SATURATED FAT)
17.6g CARBOHYDRATE
569kJ (136 CAL)
5.3g PROTEIN
4g FIBRE

CARROT DIP

PREPARATION TIME **10 MINUTES**
COOKING TIME **10 MINUTES**

1 medium carrot (120g), grated coarsely
½ cup (125ml) fresh orange juice
2 tablespoons goat milk yogurt
1 tablespoon finely chopped fresh mint
1 tablespoon dried currants
1cm piece fresh ginger (5g), grated

1 Place carrot and juice in small saucepan; cook, uncovered, over low heat, about 10 minutes or until liquid is evaporated. Cool 10 minutes.
2 Blend or process carrot mixture with yogurt; stir in mint, currants and ginger.

PER SERVING
2.2g TOTAL FAT
(1.2g SATURATED FAT)
26g CARBOHYDRATE
569kJ (136 CAL)
3.8g PROTEIN
4.4g FIBRE

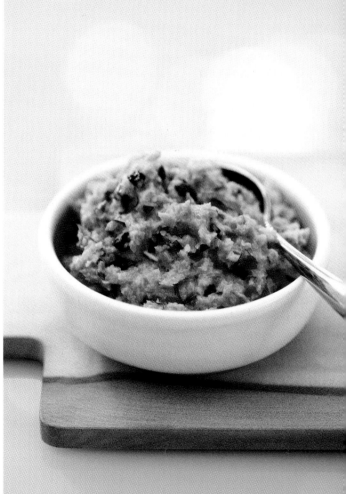

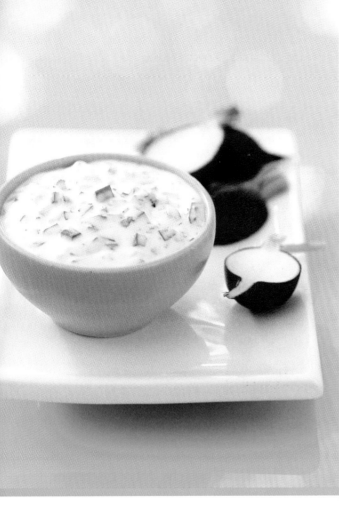

RAITA

PREPARATION TIME **10 MINUTES**

½ cup (140g) sheep milk yogurt
½ lebanese cucumber (65g), chopped finely
1 tablespoon finely chopped fresh coriander
1 clove garlic, crushed
2 teaspoons fresh lemon juice

1   Combine ingredients in small bowl.

PER SERVING
3.8g TOTAL FAT
(0g SATURATED FAT)
3.9g CARBOHYDRATE
293kJ (70 CAL)
3.2g PROTEIN
0.7g FIBRE

HUMMUS

PREPARATION TIME **5 MINUTES**
COOKING TIME **15 MINUTES**

1½ cups (375ml) water
300g can chickpeas, drained, rinsed
2 tablespoons fresh lemon juice
1 clove garlic, quartered

1   Place the water and chickpeas in small saucepan; bring to a
boil. Boil, uncovered, 10 minutes. Strain chickpeas over
small bowl; reserve ⅓ cup cooking liquid. Cool 10 minutes.
2   Blend or process chickpeas, juice and garlic with reserved
cooking liquid until just smooth.
3   Serve hummus sprinkled with finely chopped fresh flat-leaf
parsley, if desired.

PER SERVING
4.3g TOTAL FAT
(0.6g SATURATED FAT)
28.5g CARBOHYDRATE
861kJ (206 CAL)
13g PROTEIN
9.9g FIBRE

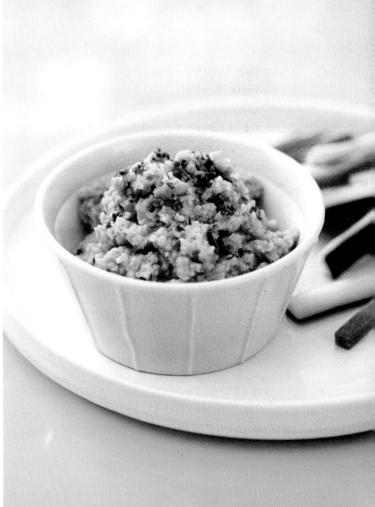

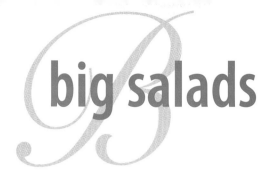
big salads

PER SERVING
9.9g TOTAL FAT
(1.3g SATURATED FAT)
15g CARBOHYDRATE
715kJ (171 CAL)
5.7g PROTEIN
5.6g FIBRE

GREEN VEGETABLE SALAD WITH AMERICAN MUSTARD DRESSING

PREPARATION TIME **10 MINUTES** COOKING TIME **10 MINUTES** SERVES **1**

50g green beans, trimmed

50g snow peas, trimmed

50g sugar snap peas, trimmed

¼ cup loosely packed fresh flat-leaf parsley leaves

2 tablespoons fresh chervil leaves

1 cup (25g) baby rocket leaves

1 tablespoon dried currants

AMERICAN MUSTARD DRESSING
2 teaspoons american mustard

2 teaspoons fresh lemon juice

2 teaspoons olive oil

1 Boil, steam or microwave beans and peas, separately, until just tender; drain. Rinse beans and peas under cold water; drain.
2 Meanwhile, place ingredients for american mustard dressing in screw-top jar; shake well.
3 Place beans and peas in medium bowl with herbs, rocket and currants; toss gently to combine.
4 Serve salad drizzled with dressing.

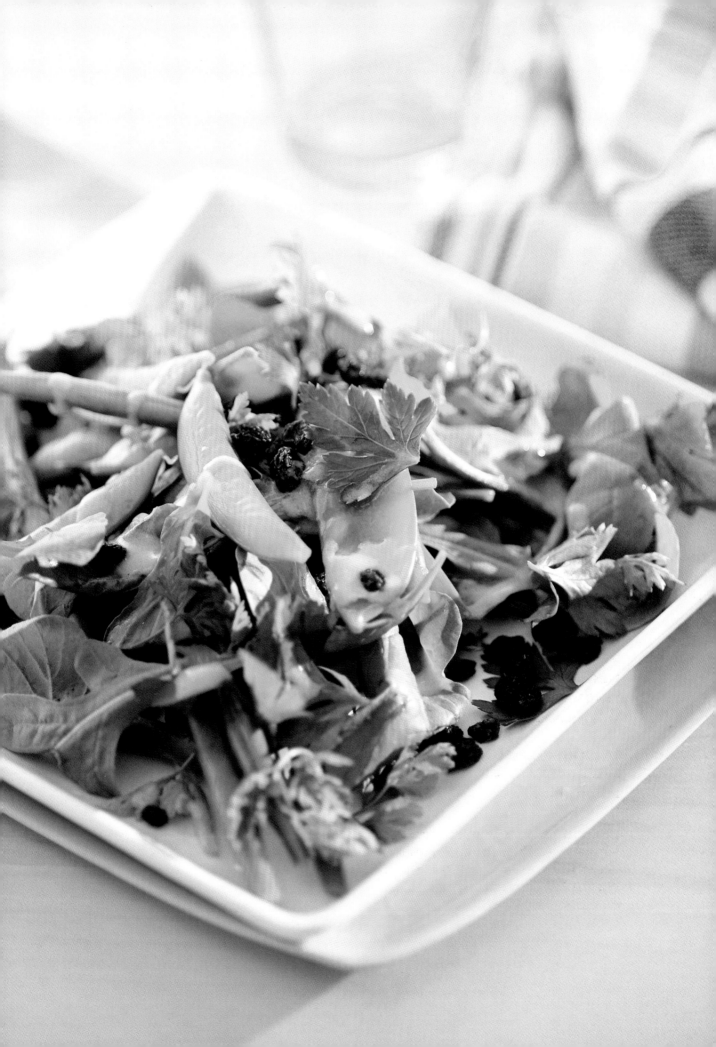

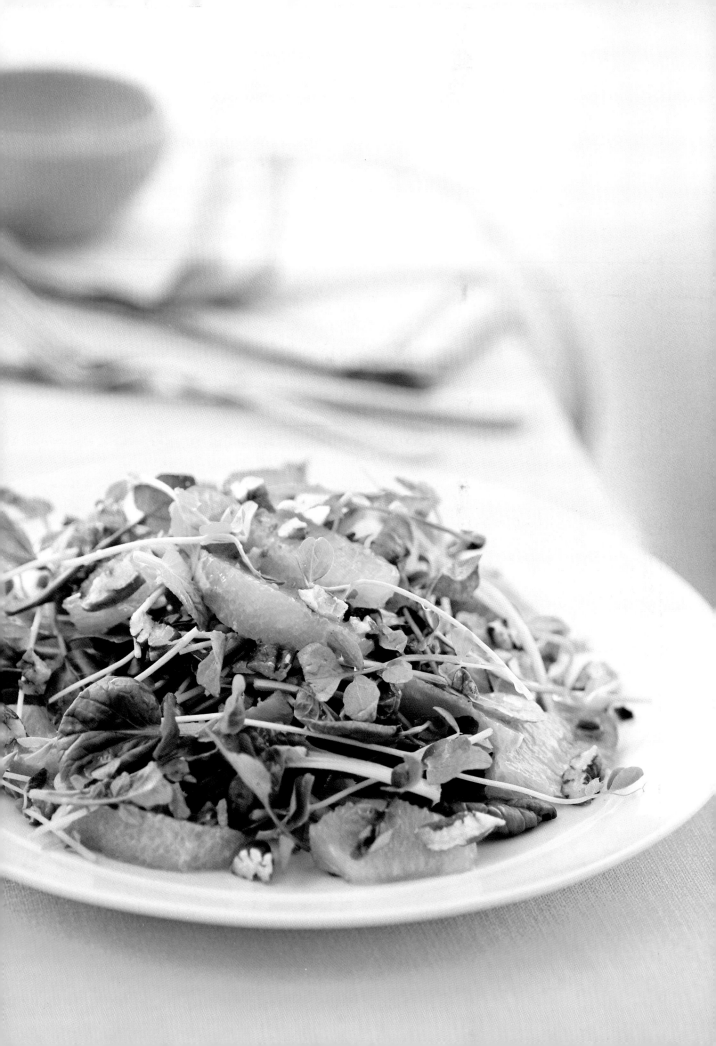

PER SERVING
42.1g TOTAL FAT
(**3.4g** SATURATED FAT)
29.8g CARBOHYDRATE
2241kJ (536 CAL)
10.6g PROTEIN
11.6g FIBRE

LAMB'S LETTUCE SALAD WITH PECANS AND ORANGE

PREPARATION TIME **10 MINUTES** SERVES **1**

Lamb's lettuce, also known as mâche or corn salad, has a mild, almost nutty, flavour and tender, narrow, dark green leaves. You need a 225g punnet for this recipe. It is available from most greengrocers.

20g watercress

25g lamb's lettuce

30g snow pea sprouts, trimmed

⅓ cup (45g) toasted pecans, chopped coarsely

2 teaspoons olive oil

2 small oranges (360g)

1 Place watercress, lettuce, sprouts, nuts and oil in medium bowl.
2 Segment oranges over salad to save juice. Add orange segments to bowl; toss gently to combine.

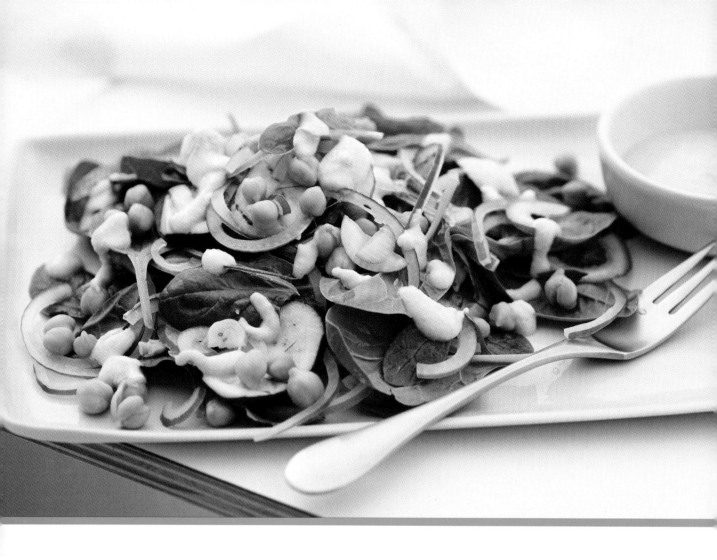

ORANGE, FENNEL AND ALMOND SALAD

PREPARATION TIME **10 MINUTES** COOKING TIME **10 MINUTES** SERVES **1**

PER SERVING
20.8g TOTAL FAT
(1.5g SATURATED FAT)
26.5g CARBOHYDRATE
1363kJ (326 CAL)
8.5g PROTEIN
9.6g FIBRE

⅓ cup (80ml) fresh orange juice

2 teaspoons almond oil

1 baby fennel bulb (130g)

1 large orange (300g), segmented

50g baby spinach leaves

¼ cup (20g) flaked almonds

1   Place juice in small saucepan; bring to a boil. Boil, uncovered, until juice reduces to
    1 tablespoon; cool 10 minutes. Combine juice with oil in small jug.
2   Meanwhile, reserve fennel tips from fennel; slice fennel thinly.
3   Place fennel in medium bowl with orange, spinach and nuts; toss gently to combine.
4   Serve salad drizzled with dressing and sprinkled with fennel tips.

SPINACH AND ZUCCHINI SALAD
WITH YOGURT HUMMUS

PREPARATION TIME **25 MINUTES** (PLUS STANDING TIME) COOKING TIME **30 MINUTES** SERVES **1**

½ cup (100g) dried chickpeas

1 small zucchini (90g), sliced thickly

1 clove garlic, unpeeled

2 tablespoons fresh lemon juice

2 teaspoons tahini

1 tablespoon goat milk yogurt

60g baby spinach leaves

½ small red onion (50g), sliced thinly

PER SERVING
14.6g TOTAL FAT
(**2.3g** SATURATED FAT)
43.4g CARBOHYDRATE
1701kJ (407 CAL)
24.3g PROTEIN
18.8g FIBRE

1 Place chickpeas in small bowl, cover with water; stand overnight, drain. Rinse under cold water; drain.
2 Cook chickpeas in small saucepan of boiling water, uncovered, until just tender; drain over small bowl, reserve 2 teaspoons of the liquid. Rinse chickpeas under cold water; drain.
3 Meanwhile, cook zucchini and garlic on heated lightly oiled grill plate (or grill or barbecue) until browned both sides. When cool enough to handle, peel garlic.
4 Blend or process ¼ cup cooked chickpeas, juice, tahini, yogurt, reserved liquid and garlic until smooth.
5 Place spinach, onion and remaining chickpeas in medium bowl; toss gently to combine.
6 Serve salad drizzled with yogurt hummus.

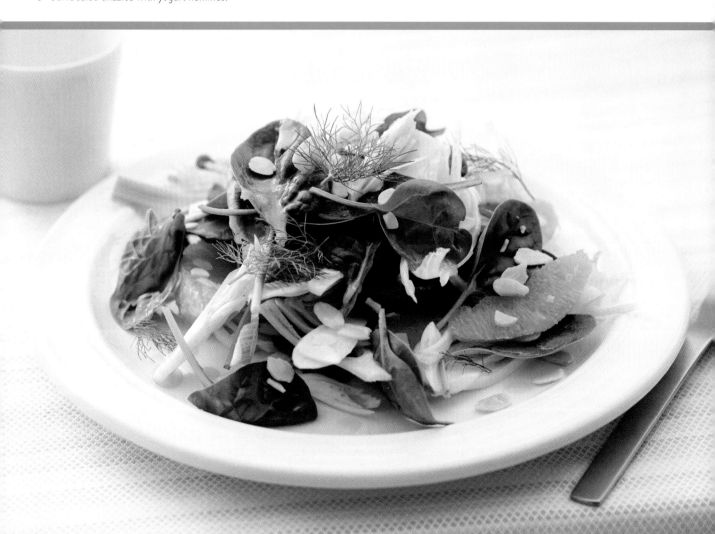

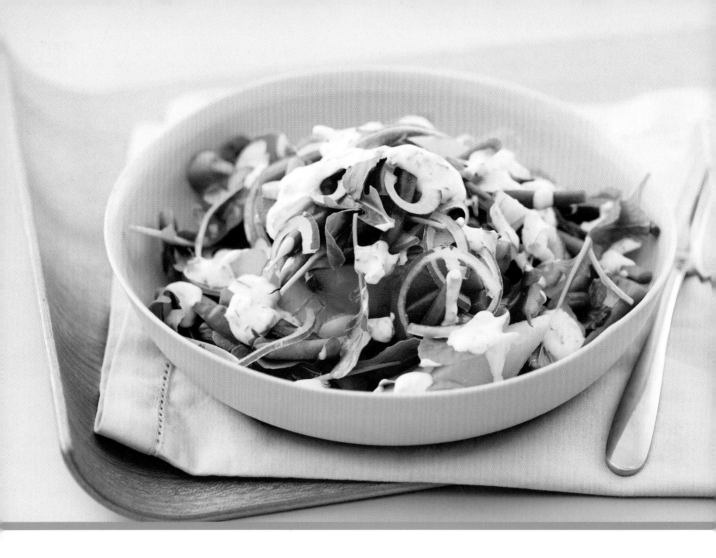

GREEK SALAD

PREPARATION TIME **10 MINUTES** SERVES **1**

PER SERVING
18.1g TOTAL FAT
(6.6g SATURATED FAT)
19.5g CARBOHYDRATE
1196kJ (286 CAL)
11.3g PROTEIN
6.5g FIBRE

½ **baby cos lettuce (90g), leaves separated**

1 **medium tomato (150g), cut into thick wedges**

½ **small red capsicum (75g), chopped coarsely**

1 **lebanese cucumber (130g), chopped coarsely**

¼ **cup (40g) seeded kalamata olives**

50g **goat milk fetta, crumbled**

2 **teaspoons fresh lemon juice**

2 **teaspoons olive oil**

1 Place ingredients in large bowl; toss gently to combine.

POTATO AND BEAN SALAD WITH LEMON YOGURT DRESSING

PREPARATION TIME **15 MINUTES** COOKING TIME **15 MINUTES** SERVES **1**

2 small potatoes (240g), unpeeled, cut into wedges

150g green beans, trimmed, cut into 3cm lengths

1 cup (230g) baby rocket leaves

½ small red onion (50g), sliced thinly

LEMON YOGURT DRESSING

⅓ cup (95g) sheep milk yogurt

1 teaspoon finely grated lemon rind

1 tablespoon fresh lemon juice

1 tablespoon finely chopped fresh flat-leaf parsley

PER SERVING
6.6g TOTAL FAT
(**1g** SATURATED FAT)
43.9g CARBOHYDRATE
1308kJ (313 CAL)
15.2g PROTEIN
10.3g FIBRE

1 Boil, steam or microwave potato and beans, separately, until tender; drain. Rinse beans under cold water; drain.
2 Meanwhile, combine ingredients for lemon yogurt dressing in small bowl.
3 Place potato and beans in medium bowl with rocket and onion; toss gently to combine. Serve salad drizzled with dressing.

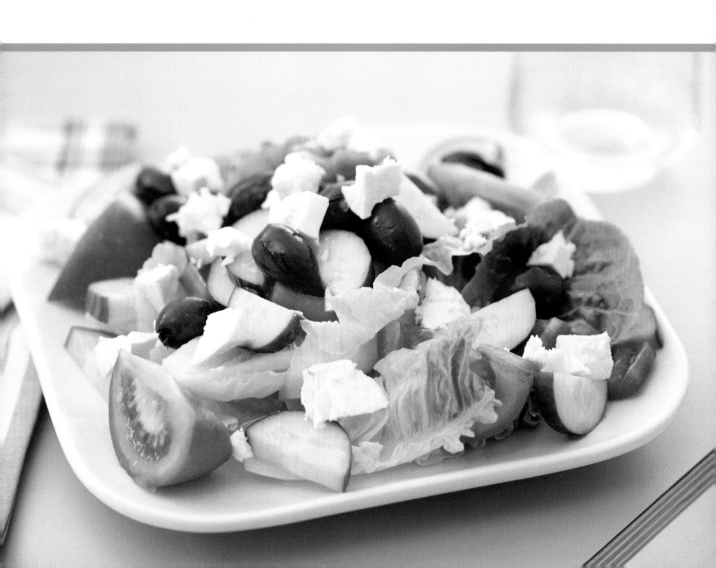

PER SERVING
7.4g TOTAL FAT
(**1g** SATURATED FAT)
11.9g CARBOHYDRATE
798kJ (191 CAL)
17.5g PROTEIN
10.3g FIBRE

PAN-FRIED TOFU WITH VIETNAMESE COLESLAW SALAD

PREPARATION TIME **20 MINUTES** COOKING TIME **5 MINUTES** SERVES **1**

100g firm silken tofu

1 small carrot (70g)

½ cup (40g) finely shredded green cabbage

½ cup (40g) finely shredded red cabbage

½ small yellow capsicum (75g), sliced thinly

½ cup (40g) bean sprouts

2 green onions, sliced thinly

¼ cup loosely packed fresh coriander leaves

LIME AND GARLIC DRESSING
¼ cup (60ml) fresh lime juice

1 clove garlic, crushed

1. Place tofu, in single layer, on absorbent-paper-lined tray; cover tofu with more absorbent paper, stand 10 minutes.
2. Meanwhile, using vegetable peeler, slice carrot into ribbons. Place in medium bowl with cabbages, capsicum, sprouts, onion and coriander; toss gently to combine.
3. Place ingredients for lime and garlic dressing in screw-top jar; shake well.
4. Cut tofu into four slices; cook tofu in heated lightly oiled small frying pan until browned both sides.
5. Drizzle dressing over salad; serve with tofu.

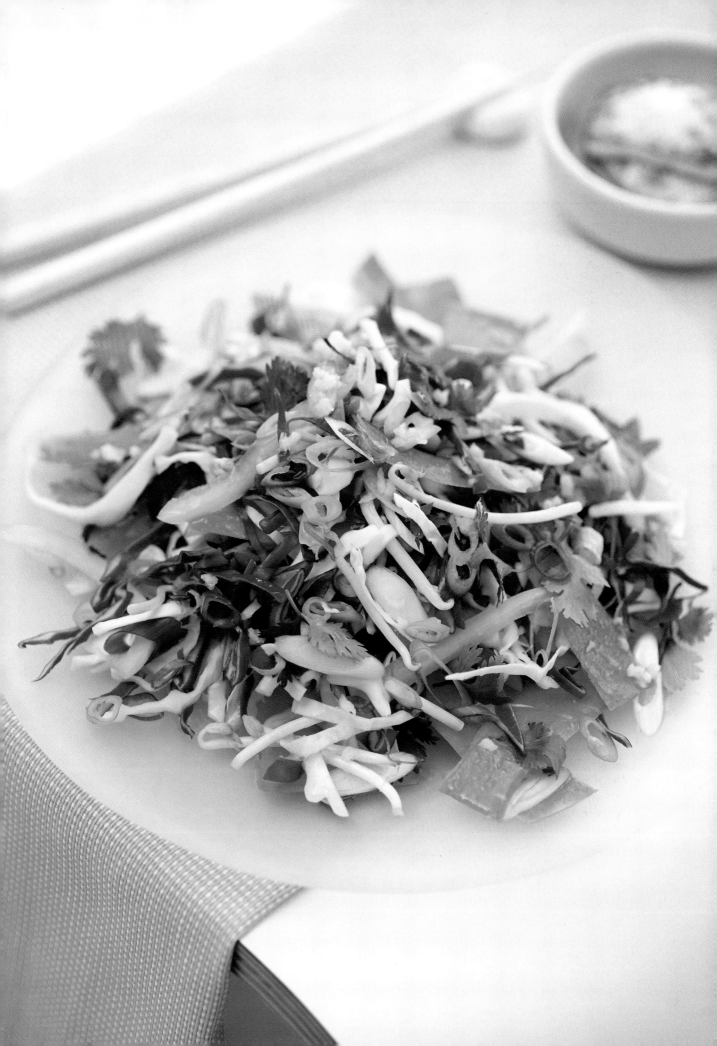

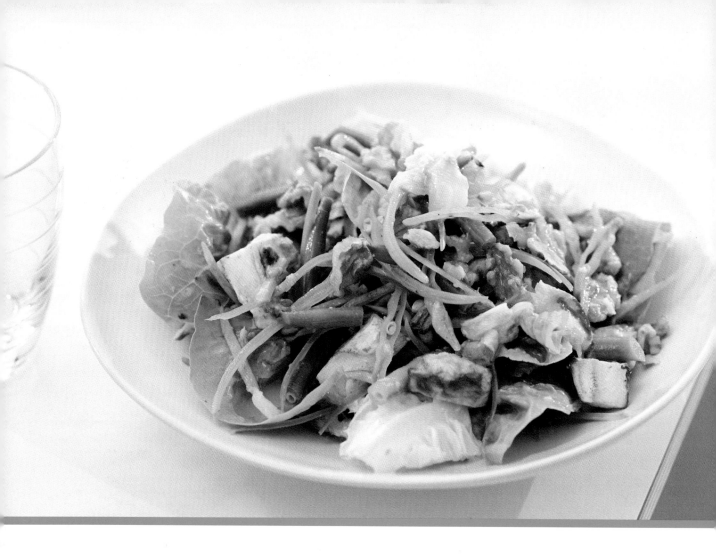

PEARL BARLEY SALAD

PREPARATION TIME **10 MINUTES** COOKING TIME **25 MINUTES** SERVES **1**

PER SERVING
2.9g TOTAL FAT
(0.4g SATURATED FAT)
68.4g CARBOHYDRATE
1513kJ (362 CAL)
13.5g PROTEIN
17g FIBRE

½ cup (100g) pearl barley

125g asparagus, trimmed, cut into 4cm lengths

125g cherry tomatoes, halved

½ lebanese cucumber (65g), sliced thinly

¾ cup (45g) finely shredded iceberg lettuce

2 tablespoons coarsely chopped fresh basil

2 tablespoons fresh lemon juice

1   Cook barley in small saucepan of boiling water, uncovered, about 25 minutes or until tender;
    drain. Cool 10 minutes.
2   Meanwhile, boil, steam or microwave asparagus until just tender; drain.
3   Place barley and asparagus in medium bowl with remaining ingredients; toss gently to combine.

COS, SNOW PEA AND ROASTED CELERIAC SALAD

PREPARATION TIME **15 MINUTES** COOKING TIME **20 MINUTES** SERVES **1**

100g celeriac, chopped coarsely

4 cloves garlic, unpeeled

cooking-oil spray

50g baby green beans, trimmed, chopped coarsely

2 tablespoons fresh lemon juice

2 teaspoons walnut oil

½ baby cos lettuce (90g), torn

50g snow peas, trimmed, sliced thinly

½ cup (50g) toasted walnuts, chopped coarsely

PER SERVING
46.9g TOTAL FAT
(13.2g SATURATED FAT)
14g CARBOHYDRATE
2215kJ (530 CAL)
13.7g PROTEIN
14.1g FIBRE

1 Preheat oven to very hot (240°C/220°C fan-forced).
2 Place celeriac and garlic on shallow oven tray; spray with oil. Roast, uncovered, about 20 minutes or until celeriac is just tender and garlic softens.
3 Meanwhile, boil, steam or microwave beans until tender; drain. Rinse under cold water; drain.
4 When garlic is cool enough to handle, squeeze garlic from skins into screw-top jar. Add juice and oil; shake well.
5 Place celeriac and beans in medium bowl with lettuce, snow peas, nuts and dressing; toss gently to combine.

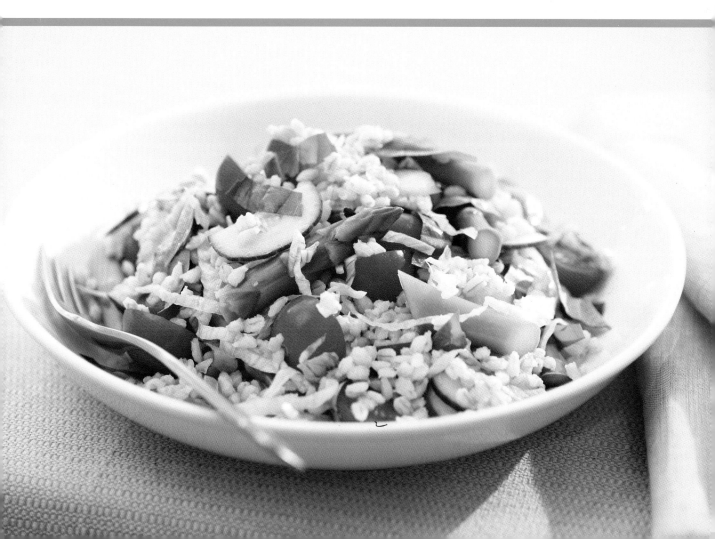

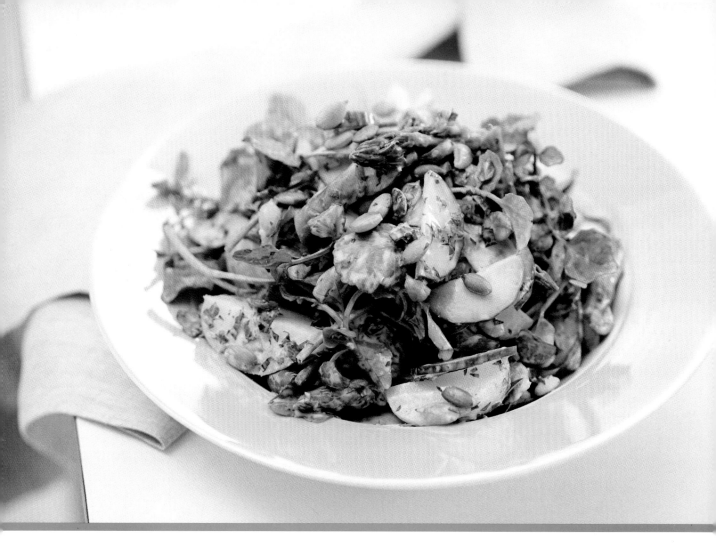

CHICKPEA, WATERCRESS AND CAPSICUM SALAD

PREPARATION TIME **15 MINUTES** (PLUS STANDING TIME) COOKING TIME **30 MINUTES** SERVES **1**

PER SERVING
21.4g TOTAL FAT
(1.5g SATURATED FAT)
15.8g CARBOHYDRATE
1371kJ (328 CAL)
16g PROTEIN
11.4g FIBRE

¼ cup (50g) dried chickpeas

100g watercress

1 tablespoon water

1 clove garlic, quartered

¼ cup (35g) toasted slivered almonds

¼ cup (60ml) fresh lemon juice

⅓ small red capsicum (50g), sliced thinly

⅓ small yellow capsicum (50g), sliced thinly

1 Place chickpeas in small bowl, cover with water; stand overnight, drain. Rinse under cold water; drain.
2 Cook chickpeas in small saucepan of boiling water, uncovered, until just tender; drain. Rinse under cold water; drain.
3 Trim watercress; reserve stalks. Blend or process watercress stalks with the water, garlic, a third of the chickpeas, 1 tablespoon of the nuts and 2 tablespoons of the juice until smooth. Transfer to medium bowl; stir in remaining chickpeas and remaining nuts.
4 Place watercress leaves and capsicums in medium bowl with remaining juice; toss gently to combine. Top with chickpea mixture.

POTATO AND ASPARAGUS SALAD
WITH YOGURT AND MINT DRESSING

PREPARATION TIME **20 MINUTES** COOKING TIME **20 MINUTES** SERVES **1**

150g baby new potatoes, unpeeled

125g asparagus, trimmed, cut into 3cm lengths

½ lebanese cucumber (65g), sliced thinly

40g watercress, trimmed

¼ cup (40g) toasted pepitas

YOGURT AND MINT DRESSING

2 tablespoons sheep milk yogurt

1 teaspoon finely grated lime rind

2 teaspoons fresh lime juice

¼ cup finely chopped fresh mint

PER SERVING
16.8g TOTAL FAT
(**1g** SATURATED FAT)
25.7g CARBOHYDRATE
1672kJ (400 CAL)
10.7g PROTEIN
11.8g FIBRE

1 Boil, steam or microwave potatoes until tender; drain. When cool enough to handle, quarter potatoes.
2 Meanwhile, boil, steam or microwave asparagus until tender; drain. Rinse under cold water; drain.
3 Combine ingredients for yogurt and mint dressing in small bowl.
4 Place potato and asparagus in medium bowl with cucumber, watercress, pepitas and dressing; toss gently to combine.

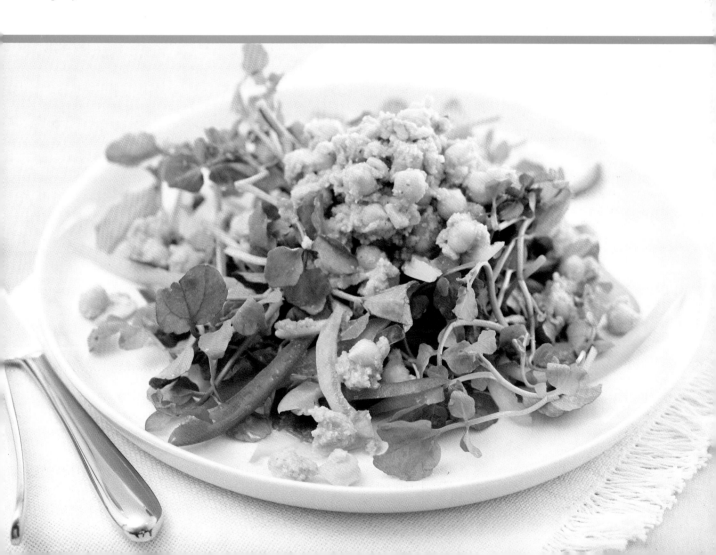

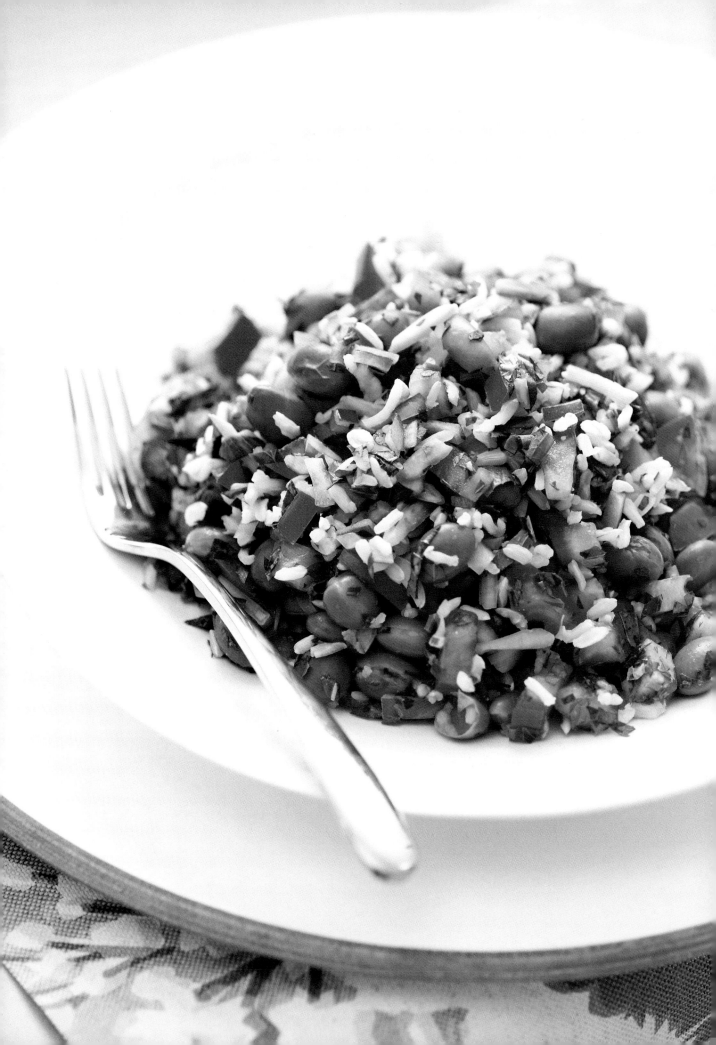

PER SERVING
18.4g TOTAL FAT
(2.1g SATURATED FAT)
63.4g CARBOHYDRATE
2140kJ (512 CAL)
21.3g PROTEIN
13.4g FIBRE

BORLOTTI BEAN, BROWN RICE AND ALMOND SALAD

PREPARATION TIME **10 MINUTES** (PLUS STANDING TIME) COOKING TIME **20 MINUTES** SERVES **1**

¼ **cup (50g) dried borlotti beans**

¼ **cup (50g) brown long-grain rice**

½ **small red onion (50g), chopped finely**

¼ **cup finely chopped fresh flat-leaf parsley**

¼ **cup finely chopped fresh mint**

1 medium tomato (150g), chopped finely

1 tablespoon toasted slivered almonds

2 tablespoons fresh lemon juice

2 teaspoons olive oil

1 Place beans in small bowl, cover with water; stand overnight, drain. Rinse under cold water; drain.
2 Cook beans in small saucepan of boiling water, uncovered, until just tender; drain. Rinse under cold water; drain.
3 Meanwhile, cook rice in small saucepan of boiling water, uncovered, until rice is tender; drain. Rinse under cold water; drain.
4 Place beans and rice in medium bowl with remaining ingredients; toss gently to combine.

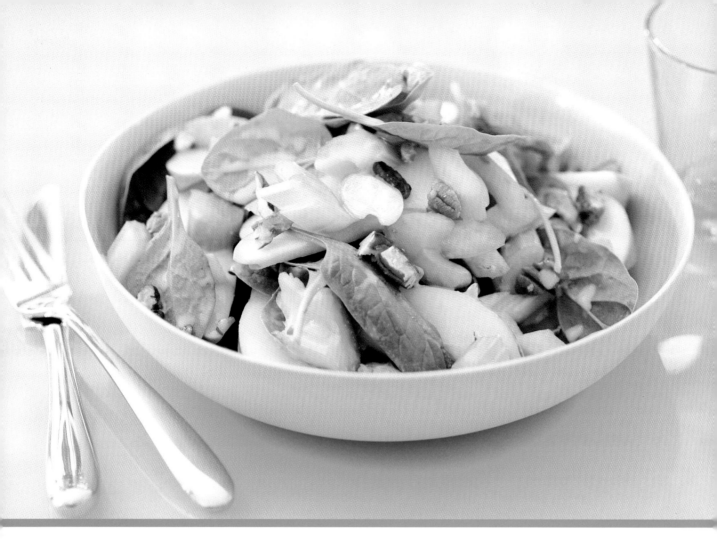

ROASTED EGG TOMATOES WITH BARLEY SALAD

PREPARATION TIME **15 MINUTES** COOKING TIME **20 MINUTES** SERVES **1**

PER SERVING
6.4g TOTAL FAT
(0.9g SATURATED FAT)
44.4g CARBOHYDRATE
1191kJ (285 CAL)
10.7g PROTEIN
13.4g FIBRE

¼ cup (50g) pearl barley

2 medium egg tomatoes (150g), cut into thick wedges

1 small green capsicum (150g), chopped finely

½ small red onion (50g), chopped finely

½ cup coarsely chopped fresh flat-leaf parsley

LEMON AND DILL DRESSING
2 tablespoons fresh lemon juice

1 tablespoon finely chopped fresh dill

1 teaspoon olive oil

1 clove garlic, crushed

1   Preheat oven to very hot (240°C/220°C fan-forced).
2   Cook barley in small saucepan of boiling water, uncovered, about 20 minutes or until just tender; drain. Rinse under cold water; drain.
3   Meanwhile, place tomato, cut-side up, on lightly oiled oven tray. Roast tomato, uncovered, about 15 minutes or until just softened.
4   Place ingredients for lemon and dill dressing in screw-top jar; shake well.
5   Place barley and half of the tomato in medium bowl with capsicum, onion, parsley and dressing; toss gently to combine. Top with remaining tomato.

PEAR, SPINACH, WALNUT AND CELERY SALAD

PREPARATION TIME **10 MINUTES** SERVES **1**

1 large pear (330g), cut into thin wedges

60g baby spinach leaves

¼ cup (25g) toasted walnuts, chopped coarsely

1 trimmed celery stalk (100g), chopped coarsely

MUSTARD DRESSING
2 teaspoons american mustard

1 teaspoon cider vinegar

1 tablespoon fresh apple juice

PER SERVING
18.1g TOTAL FAT
(**1.1g** SATURATED FAT)
50.5g CARBOHYDRATE
1601kJ (383 CAL)
6.9g PROTEIN
12.1g FIBRE

1 Place ingredients for mustard dressing in screw-top jar; shake well.
2 Place pear, spinach, nuts and celery in medium bowl; toss gently to combine.
3 Serve salad drizzled with dressing.

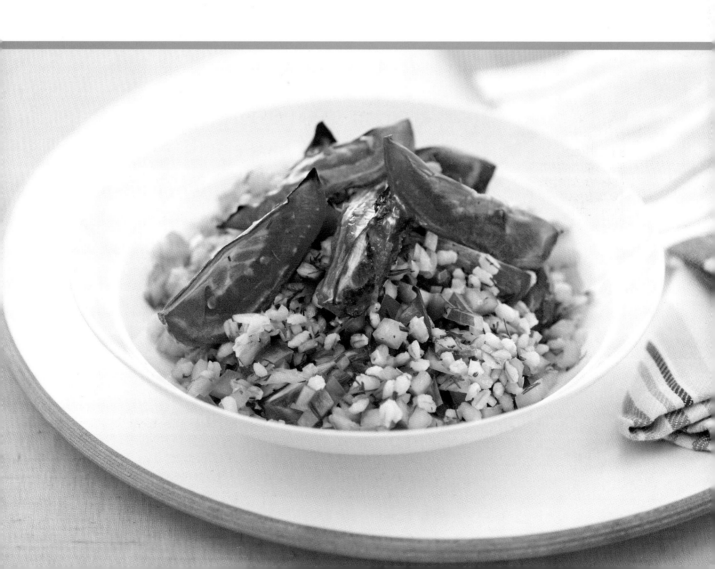

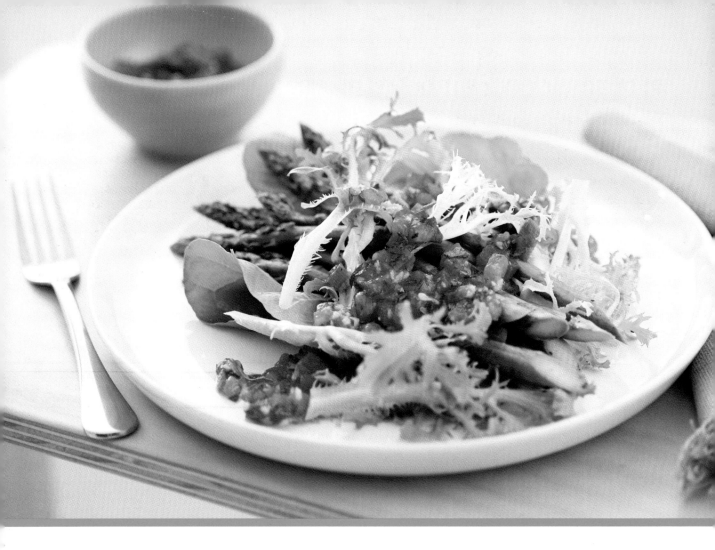

THAI SOY BEAN SALAD WITH GRAPES AND PINK GRAPEFRUIT

PREPARATION TIME **15 MINUTES** (PLUS STANDING TIME) COOKING TIME **20 MINUTES** SERVES **1**

PER SERVING
11.3g TOTAL FAT
(**1.6g** SATURATED FAT)
38.3g CARBOHYDRATE
1517kJ (363 CAL)
24.6g PROTEIN
16.9g FIBRE

¼ cup (50g) dried soya beans

1 small pink grapefruit (350g), segmented

50g green grapes, halved

1 small white onion (80g), chopped finely

50g snow pea sprouts, trimmed

¼ cup finely chopped fresh coriander

¼ cup finely chopped fresh mint

1 fresh kaffir lime leaf, shredded finely

2 tablespoons fresh lime juice

1 Place beans in small bowl, cover with water; stand overnight, drain. Rinse under cold water; drain.
2 Cook beans in small saucepan of boiling water, uncovered, until just tender; drain. Rinse under cold water; drain.
3 Place beans in medium bowl with remaining ingredients; toss gently to combine.

GRILLED ASPARAGUS WITH WARM TOMATO DRESSING

PREPARATION TIME **20 MINUTES** COOKING TIME **15 MINUTES** SERVES **1**

1 medium tomato (150g), chopped finely

1 clove garlic, crushed

2 tablespoons fresh lemon juice

1 tablespoon finely chopped fresh basil

1 tablespoon finely chopped fresh flat-leaf parsley

125g asparagus, trimmed

25g curly endive, torn

25g rocket leaves

PER SERVING
0.7g TOTAL FAT
(0g SATURATED FAT)
6.7g CARBOHYDRATE
272kJ (65 CAL)
6.3g PROTEIN
6.5g FIBRE

1 Combine tomato, garlic and juice in small saucepan; bring to a boil. Reduce heat; simmer, uncovered, 2 minutes. Remove from heat; stir in herbs.

2 Meanwhile, cook asparagus on heated lightly oiled grill plate (or grill or barbecue) until just tender.

3 Place endive and rocket on medium serving plate; top with asparagus and tomato mixture.

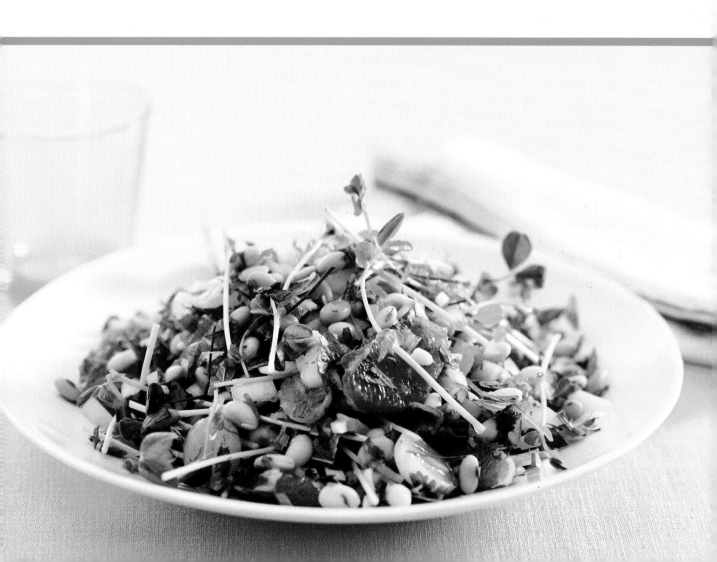

PER SERVING
12.2g TOTAL FAT
(**1.6g** SATURATED FAT)
41.5g CARBOHYDRATE
1367kJ (327 CAL)
11.1g PROTEIN
9.1g FIBRE

SOBA SALAD WITH SEAWEED, GINGER AND VEGETABLES

PREPARATION TIME **10 MINUTES** COOKING TIME **5 MINUTES** SERVES **1**

Wakame, a bright green seaweed usually sold in dried form, is used in soups, salads and seasonings. Dried wakame must be softened by soaking for about 10 minutes, and any hard stems are then discarded. It is available from most Asian food stores.
Soba is a Japanese noodle, similar in appearance to spaghetti, made from buckwheat.

5g wakame

50g soba

1 lebanese cucumber (130g), seeded, cut into matchsticks

1 small carrot (70g), cut into matchsticks

1 tablespoon toasted sesame seeds

1 green onion, sliced thinly

1cm piece fresh ginger (5g), grated

1 teaspoon sesame oil

2 tablespoons fresh lime juice

1 teaspoon tamari

1 Place wakame in small bowl, cover with cold water; stand about 10 minutes or until wakame softens, drain. Discard any hard stems; chop coarsely.
2 Meanwhile, cook soba in small saucepan of boiling water, uncovered, until just tender; drain. Rinse under cold water; drain. Chop soba coarsely.
3 Place wakame and soba in medium bowl with remaining ingredients; toss gently to combine.

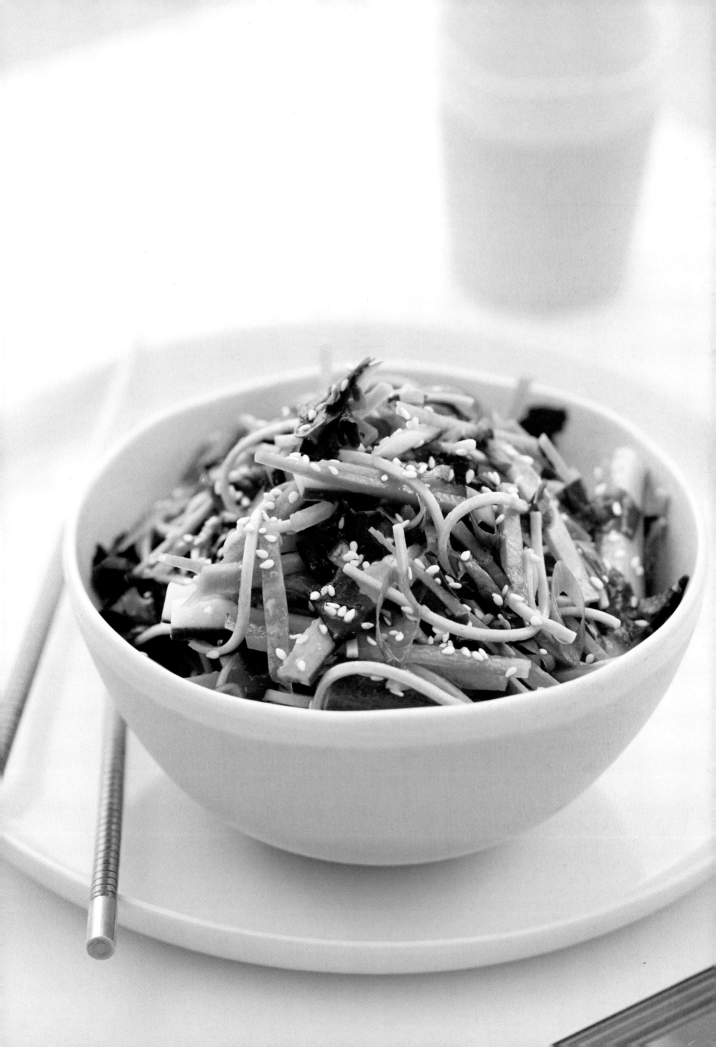

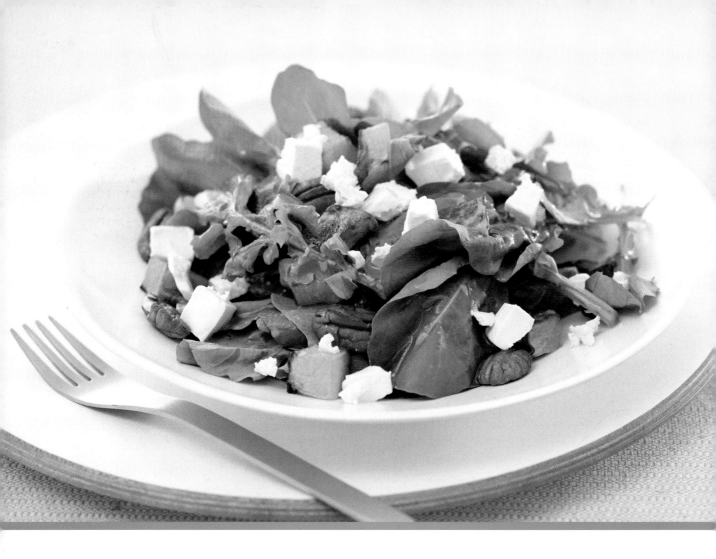

TOMATO AND AVOCADO SALAD WITH TOFU PESTO

PREPARATION TIME **10 MINUTES** SERVES **1**

PER SERVING
40.6g TOTAL FAT
(6.4g SATURATED FAT)
7g CARBOHYDRATE
2044kJ (489 CAL)
24g PROTEIN
8.6g FIBRE

1 medium tomato (150g), cut into wedges

½ medium avocado (125g), sliced thickly

100g firm silken tofu, diced into 3cm pieces

50g mesclun

1 tablespoon fresh basil leaves

TOFU PESTO
1 tablespoon toasted pine nuts

50g firm tofu

½ cup firmly packed fresh basil leaves

1 tablespoon fresh lemon juice

1 tablespoon water

1 Blend or process ingredients for tofu pesto until smooth.
2 Combine salad ingredients in medium bowl; serve salad topped with pesto.

ROASTED PUMPKIN, PECAN AND FETTA SALAD

PREPARATION TIME **15 MINUTES** COOKING TIME **20 MINUTES** SERVES **1**

100g pumpkin, chopped coarsely

cooking-oil spray

80g rocket leaves

⅓ cup (40g) toasted pecans

50g goat fetta cheese, crumbled

CITRUS DRESSING
1 tablespoon fresh orange juice

1 tablespoon fresh lemon juice

1 teaspoon grapeseed oil

PER SERVING
44.3g TOTAL FAT
(7.9g SATURATED FAT)
12.7g CARBOHYDRATE
2111kJ (505 CAL)
14.9g PROTEIN
5.8g FIBRE

1 Preheat oven to very hot (240°C/220°C fan-forced).
2 Place pumpkin on lightly oiled oven tray; spray with oil. Roast, uncovered, about 20 minutes or until tender.
3 Place ingredients for citrus dressing in screw-top jar; shake well.
4 Combine pumpkin in medium bowl with remaining ingredients and dressing; toss gently to combine.

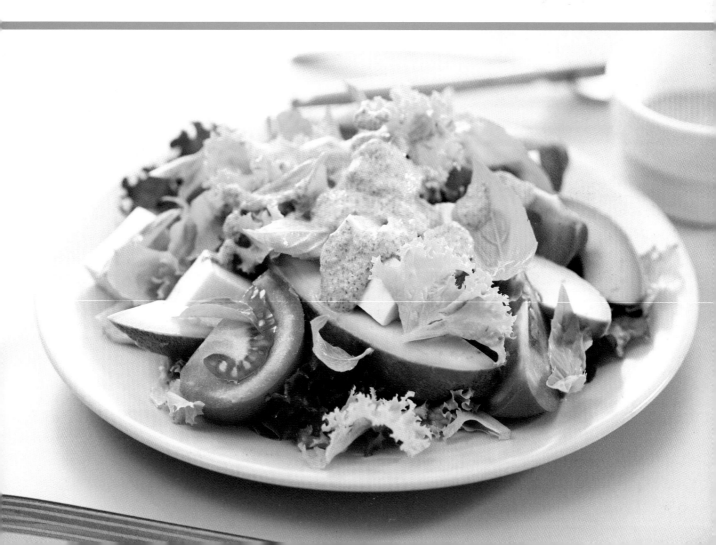

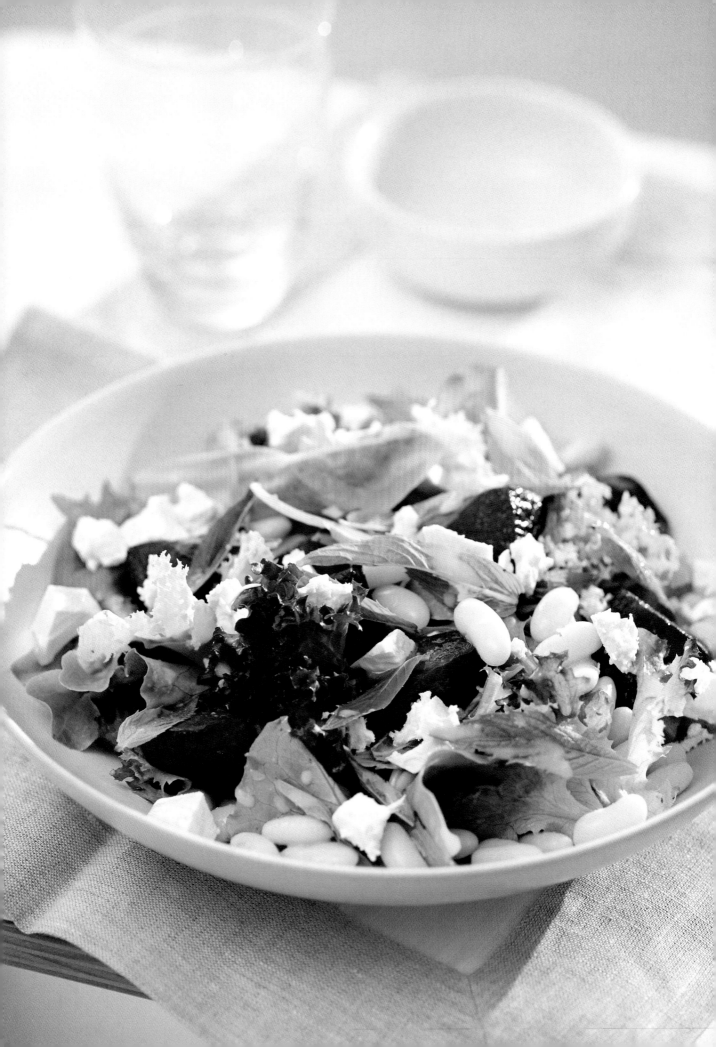

PER SERVING
10.3g TOTAL FAT
(5.4g SATURATED FAT)
39.4g CARBOHYDRATE
1417kJ (339 CAL)
21.7g PROTEIN
16.3g FIBRE

BAKED BEETROOT SALAD WITH CANNELLINI BEANS, FETTA AND MINT

PREPARATION TIME **10 MINUTES** (PLUS STANDING TIME) COOKING TIME **50 MINUTES** SERVES **1**

¼ cup (50g) dried cannellini beans

1 medium beetroot (175g), diced into 3cm pieces

cooking-oil spray

50g goat fetta cheese, crumbled

50g mesclun

¼ cup loosely packed fresh mint leaves

APPLE DRESSING
2 tablespoons fresh apple juice

2 teaspoons american mustard

1 Place beans in small bowl, cover with water; stand overnight, drain. Rinse under cold water; drain.
2 Cook beans in small saucepan of boiling water, uncovered, until just tender; drain. Rinse under cold water; drain.
3 Preheat oven to moderately hot (200°C/180°C fan-forced).
4 Place beetroot in small shallow baking dish; spray with oil. Bake, covered, about 20 minutes or until tender.
5 Place ingredients for apple dressing in screw-top jar; shake well.
6 Place beans and beetroot in medium bowl with remaining ingredients and dressing; toss gently to combine.

fruit dishes

PER SERVING
0.5g TOTAL FAT
(**0g** SATURATED FAT)
72.1g CARBOHYDRATE
1242kJ (297 CAL)
2.4g PROTEIN
9.9g FIBRE

APPLE AND PEAR COMPOTE WITH DATES

PREPARATION TIME **5 MINUTES** COOKING TIME **10 MINUTES** SERVES **1**

1 small apple (130g)

1 small pear (180g)

2 tablespoons fresh lemon juice

⅓ cup (55g) seeded coarsely chopped dried dates

1 teaspoon finely grated orange rind

2 tablespoons fresh orange juice

1 Peel and core apple and pear; dice into 2cm pieces. Combine apple and pear in small saucepan with lemon juice; cook, covered, over low heat, about 10 minutes or until fruit softens.

2 Meanwhile, combine dates, rind and orange juice in small saucepan; cook, uncovered, over low heat, stirring occasionally, about 5 minutes or until liquid is absorbed.

3 Serve compote, warm or cold, topped with date mixture and finely shredded orange rind, if desired.

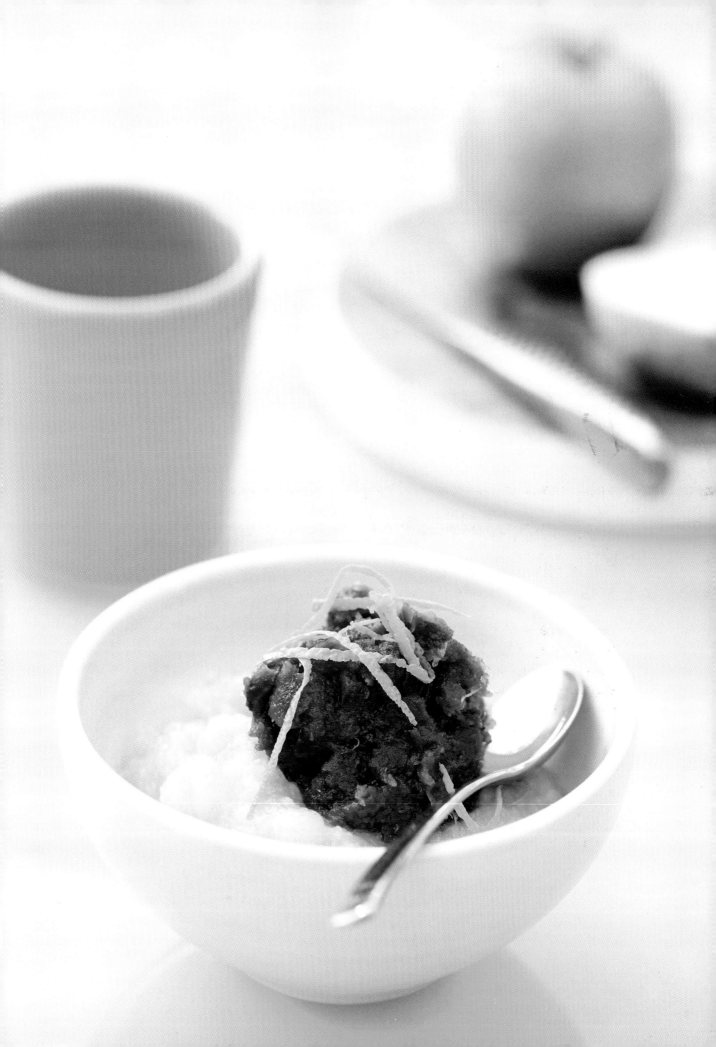

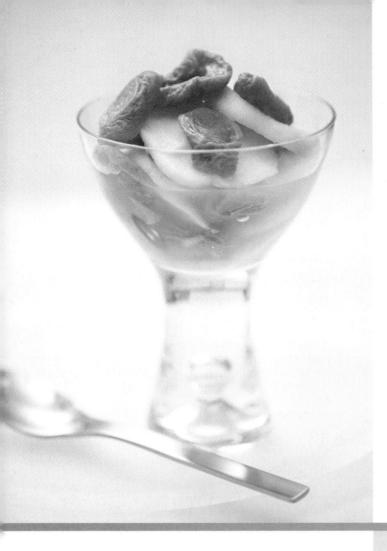

MACERATED FRUITS

PREPARATION TIME **5 MINUTES** (PLUS REFRIGERATION TIME) SERVES **1**

¼ cup (20g) dried apples
¼ cup (35g) dried apricots
½ cup (125ml) fresh apple juice
2 teaspoons fresh lemon juice

1 Combine ingredients in small bowl.
2 Cover; refrigerate 2 hours or overnight.

PER SERVING
0.2g TOTAL FAT
(**0g** SATURATED FAT)
41.4g CARBOHYDRATE
723kJ (**173 CAL**)
1.9g PROTEIN
5g FIBRE

FOUR-FRUIT COMBO

PREPARATION TIME **10 MINUTES** SERVES **1**

1 small pear (180g), chopped coarsely
1 small apple (130g), chopped coarsely
1 small pink grapefruit (350g), segmented
100g red grapes

1 Combine ingredients in medium bowl.

PER SERVING
0.8g TOTAL FAT
(**0g** SATURATED FAT)
58.5g CARBOHYDRATE
1066kJ (**255 CAL**)
4.1g PROTEIN
8.1g FIBRE

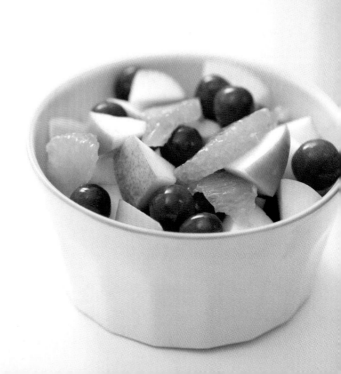

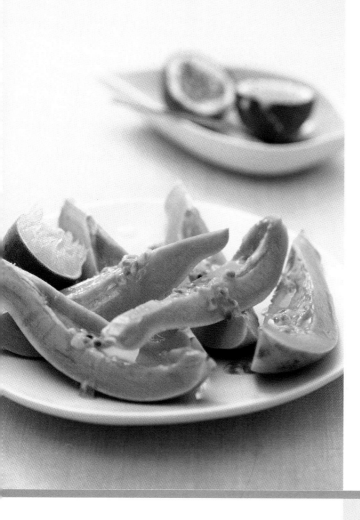

PAPAYA WITH PASSIONFRUIT AND LIME

PREPARATION TIME **10 MINUTES** SERVES **1**

We used the red-fleshed Hawaiian or Fijian variety instead of the yellow-fleshed papaya here. You need one passionfruit for this recipe.

1 small papaya (650g), cut into thick wedges

1 tablespoon fresh passionfruit pulp

2 teaspoons fresh lime juice

1 Place papaya on medium serving plate.
2 Drizzle with passionfruit and juice.

PER SERVING
0.5g TOTAL FAT
(0g SATURATED FAT)
32.3g CARBOHYDRATE
598kJ (143 CAL)
2.5g PROTEIN
13.1g FIBRE

BANANA WITH PASSIONFRUIT YOGURT

PREPARATION TIME **5 MINUTES** SERVES **1**

You need two passionfruits for this recipe.

2 tablespoons sheep milk yogurt

2 tablespoons fresh passionfruit pulp

1 medium banana (200g), sliced thickly

1 Combine yogurt and half of the passionfruit in small bowl.
2 Place banana in small bowl; top with yogurt mixture and remaining passionfruit.

PER SERVING
3.1g TOTAL FAT
(0g SATURATED FAT)
31.2g CARBOHYDRATE
757kJ (181 CAL)
5.6g PROTEIN
8.5g FIBRE

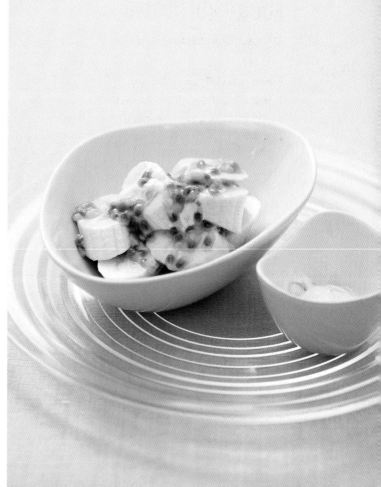

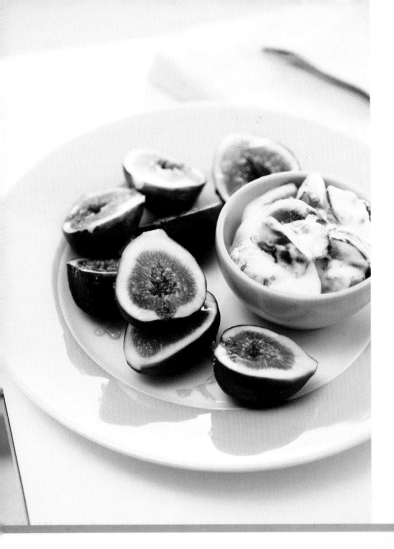

FIGS WITH SHEEP MILK YOGURT AND HONEY

PREPARATION TIME **5 MINUTES** SERVES **1**

2 medium fresh figs (120g), chopped coarsely
¼ cup (70g) sheep milk yogurt
4 medium fresh figs (240g), halved
1 teaspoon honey

1 Combine chopped figs and yogurt in small bowl.
2 Place halved figs on serving plate; drizzle with honey.
3 Serve with yogurt mixture.

PER SERVING
5.2g TOTAL FAT
(0g SATURATED FAT)
35.2g CARBOHYDRATE
932kJ (223 CAL)
7.5g PROTEIN
6.8g FIBRE

KIWI FRUIT, LYCHEE AND LIME SALAD

PREPARATION TIME **5 MINUTES** SERVES **1**

2 kiwi fruits (170g), cut into wedges
4 fresh lychees (100g)
1 tablespoon fresh mint leaves
1 tablespoon fresh lime juice

1 Combine ingredients in small bowl.

PER SERVING
0.5g TOTAL FAT
(0g SATURATED FAT)
26.8g CARBOHYDRATE
535kJ (128 CAL)
3.2g PROTEIN
6.1g FIBRE

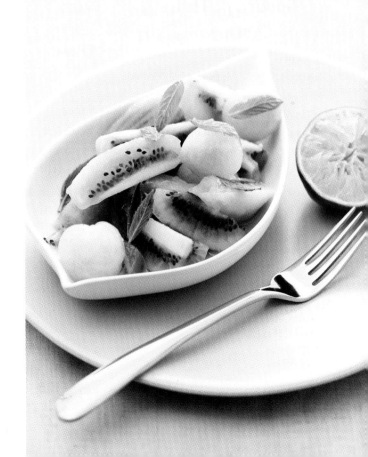

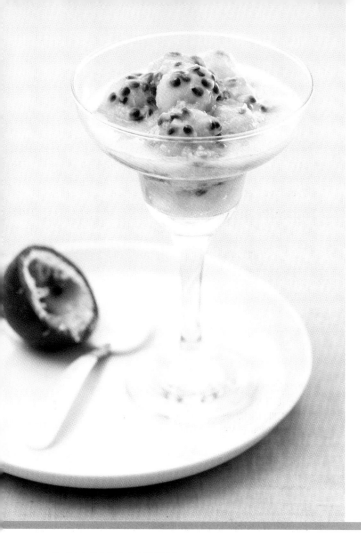

LYCHEES WITH PASSIONFRUIT

PREPARATION TIME **5 MINUTES** SERVES **1**

You need one passionfruit for this recipe.

20 fresh lychees (500g)
2 tablespoons fresh passionfruit pulp

1 Blend or process half of the lychees until smooth; stir in half of the passionfruit.
2 Place remaining lychees in small bowl; top with lychee mixture and remaining passionfruit.

PER SERVING
0.4g TOTAL FAT
(0g SATURATED FAT)
62g CARBOHYDRATE
1112kJ (266 CAL)
4.8g PROTEIN
7.8g FIBRE

BANANA WITH PASSIONFRUIT

PREPARATION TIME **5 MINUTES** SERVES **1**

You need one passionfruit for this recipe.

2 medium bananas (400g)
1 tablespoon fresh passionfruit pulp

1 Cut bananas in half lengthways; cut each half into two pieces.
2 Place banana in medium serving bowl; drizzle with passionfruit pulp.

PER SERVING
0.3g TOTAL FAT
(0g SATURATED FAT)
54.5g CARBOHYDRATE
999kJ (239 CAL)
5.2g PROTEIN
8.8g FIBRE

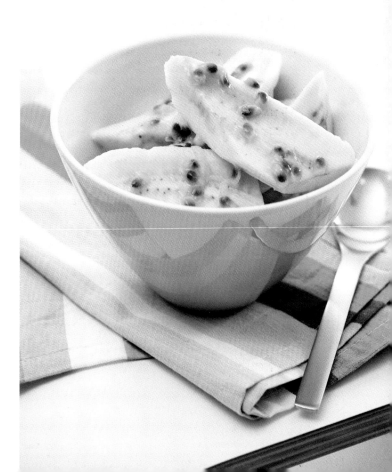

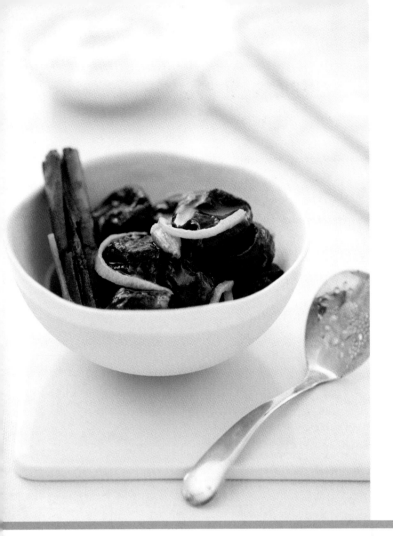

STEWED PRUNES WITH ORANGE

PREPARATION TIME **5 MINUTES** COOKING TIME **15 MINUTES** SERVES **1**

½ cup (85g) seeded dried prunes
¼ cup (60ml) fresh orange juice
¼ cup (60ml) water
5cm strip orange rind, sliced thinly
1 cinnamon stick
2 cardamon pods, bruised

1 Place ingredients in small saucepan; bring to a boil. Reduce heat; simmer, covered, 10 minutes.
2 Serve stewed prunes with sheep milk yogurt, if desired.

PER SERVING
0.4g TOTAL FAT
(0g SATURATED FAT)
42.2g CARBOHYDRATE
752kJ (180 CAL)
2.3g PROTEIN
6.8g FIBRE

BLOOD PLUMS WITH HONEY AND CARDAMON YOGURT

PREPARATION TIME **5 MINUTES** SERVES **1**

¼ cup (70g) sheep milk yogurt
2 teaspoons honey
¼ teaspoon ground cardamom
2 small blood plums (180g), quartered

1 Combine yogurt, honey and cardamom in small bowl.
2 Place plums on small serving plate; drizzle with yogurt mixture.

PER SERVING
4.4g TOTAL FAT
(0g SATURATED FAT)
26.7g CARBOHYDRATE
732kJ (175 CAL)
4.2g PROTEIN
3.6g FIBRE

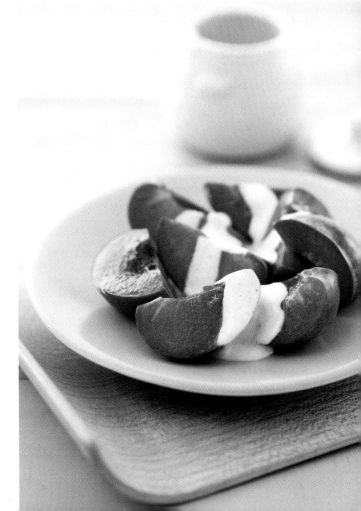

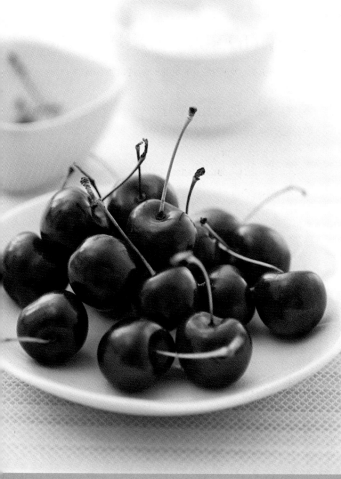

CHERRIES AND YOGURT

PREPARATION TIME **5 MINUTES** SERVES **1**

1½ cups (225g) cherries
⅓ cup (95g) sheep milk yogurt

1 Place cherries on small serving plate; serve with yogurt.

PER SERVING
6g TOTAL FAT
(0g SATURATED FAT)
23.4g CARBOHYDRATE
757kJ (181 CAL)
6g PROTEIN
2.7g FIBRE

MANGO CHEEKS
WITH LIME WEDGES

PREPARATION TIME **5 MINUTES** SERVES 1

1 large mango (600g)
½ lime, cut into wedges

1 Slice cheeks from mango; score each cheek in shallow criss-cross pattern, taking care not to cut through skin.
2 Serve mango cheeks with lime wedges.

PER SERVING
1g TOTAL FAT
(0g SATURATED FAT)
54.6g CARBOHYDRATE
1074kJ (257 CAL)
4.9g PROTEIN
8g FIBRE

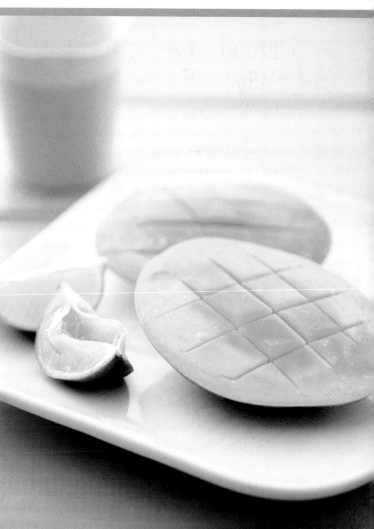

drinks & nightcaps

PER 250ML
0g TOTAL FAT
(**0g** SATURATED FAT)
1.5g CARBOHYDRATE
33kJ (8 CAL)
0.3g PROTEIN
0.4g FIBRE

PER 250ML
0.1g TOTAL FAT
(**0g** SATURATED FAT)
0.9g CARBOHYDRATE
38kJ (9 CAL)
0.2g PROTEIN
0g FIBRE

HOT GRAPEFRUIT WATER

PREPARATION TIME **5 MINUTES** MAKES **1 LITRE**

3½ cups (875ml) boiling water
½ cup (125ml) fresh grapefruit juice

1   Place the water in large jug; stir in juice.

HOT LEMON WATER

PREPARATION TIME **5 MINUTES** MAKES **1 LITRE**

3½ cups (875ml) boiling water
½ cup (125ml) fresh lemon juice

1   Place the water in large jug; stir in juice.
2   Serve with lemon slices, if desired.

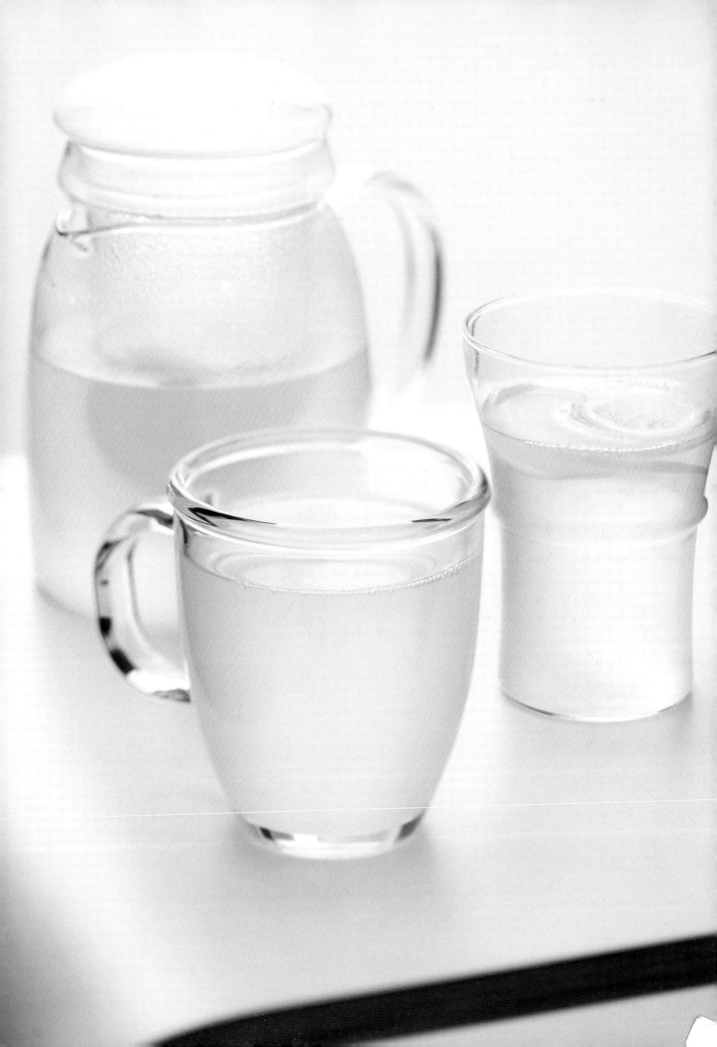

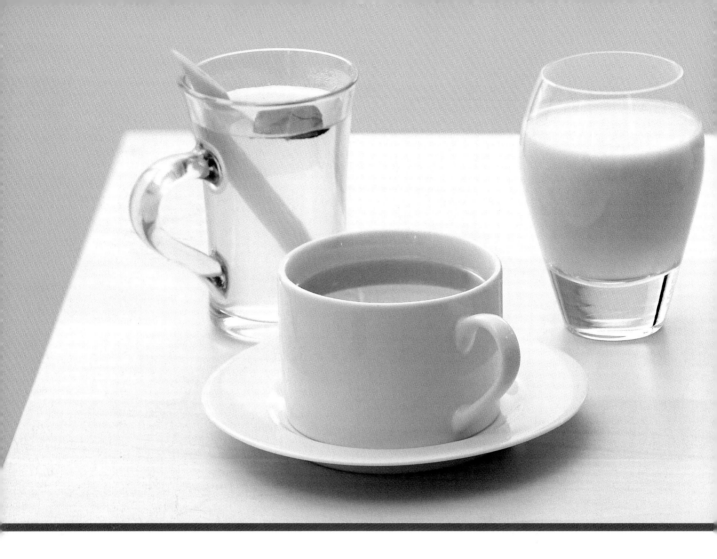

LEMON GRASS AND KAFFIR LIME TEA

PREPARATION TIME **5 MINUTES**

COOKING TIME **10 MINUTES** MAKES **1 LITRE**

10cm stick (20g) finely chopped fresh lemon grass

4 fresh kaffir lime leaves

1 litre (4 cups) water

1 Combine ingredients in small saucepan; bring to a boil.
2 Reduce heat; simmer, uncovered, 5 minutes. Cool 5 minutes; strain.

PER 250ML
0g TOTAL FAT
(**0g** SATURATED FAT)
0g CARBOHYDRATE
1kJ (0.3 CAL)
0g PROTEIN
0g FIBRE

CARDAMOM AND CHAMOMILE TEA

PREPARATION TIME **5 MINUTES**

COOKING TIME **10 MINUTES** MAKES **1 LITRE**

2 tablespoons loose-leafed chamomile tea

4 cardamom pods, bruised

1 litre (4 cups) water

1 Combine ingredients in small saucepan; bring to a boil.
2 Reduce heat; simmer, uncovered, 5 minutes. Cool 5 minutes; strain.

PER 250ML
0g TOTAL FAT
(**0g** SATURATED FAT)
0g CARBOHYDRATE
0.6kJ (0.2 CAL)
0g PROTEIN
0g FIBRE

ALMOND MILK

PREPARATION TIME **5 MINUTES**

(PLUS REFRIGERATION TIME) MAKES **¾ CUP**

1 cup (250ml) water

½ cup (70g) toasted slivered almonds

3 drops vanilla extract

1 Blend or process the water and nuts until pureed.
2 Strain mixture through muslin-lined sieve into small jug; discard solids. Add extract; stir to combine. Refrigerate until chilled.

PER 180ML
38.1g TOTAL FAT
(**3.8g** SATURATED FAT)
3.1g CARBOHYDRATE
1697kJ (406 CAL)
14.3g PROTEIN
6.3g FIBRE

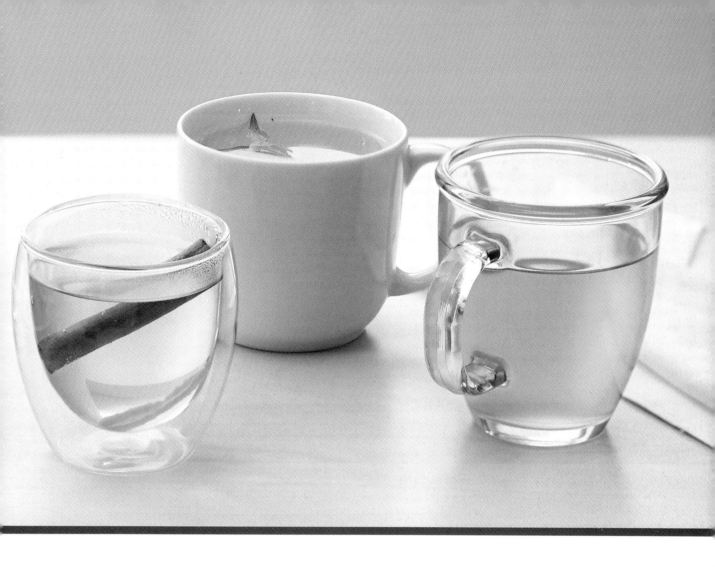

CINNAMON AND ORANGE TEA

PREPARATION TIME **5 MINUTES**

COOKING TIME **10 MINUTES** MAKES **1 LITRE**

2 cinnamon sticks
10cm strip orange rind
1 litre (4 cups) water

1 Combine ingredients in small saucepan; bring to a boil.
2 Reduce heat; simmer, uncovered, 5 minutes. Cool 5 minutes; strain.

PER 250ML
0g TOTAL FAT
(**0g** SATURATED FAT)
0.6g CARBOHYDRATE
13kJ (3 CAL)
0.1g PROTEIN
0.2g FIBRE

MINT TEA

PREPARATION TIME **5 MINUTES**

MAKES **1 LITRE**

½ cup coarsely chopped fresh mint
1 litre (4 cups) boiling water

1 Combine ingredients in large heatproof jug.
2 Stand, uncovered, 3 minutes; strain.

tip Any unused tea can be reheated in a microwave oven or served chilled.

PER 250ML
0.1g TOTAL FAT
(**0g** SATURATED FAT)
0.3g CARBOHYDRATE
13kJ (3 CAL)
0.2g PROTEIN
0.5g FIBRE

GINGER TEA

PREPARATION TIME **5 MINUTES**

COOKING TIME **20 MINUTES** MAKES **1 LITRE**

20cm piece fresh ginger (100g), sliced thinly
1.5 litres (6 cups) water

1 Combine ingredients in medium saucepan; bring to a boil.
2 Reduce heat; simmer, uncovered, about 15 minutes or until liquid has reduced by a third. Cool 5 minutes; strain.

tip Any unused tea can be reheated in a microwave oven or served chilled.

PER 250ML
0.1g TOTAL FAT
(**0g** SATURATED FAT)
1g CARBOHYDRATE
29kJ (7 CAL)
0.2g PROTEIN
0.7g FIBRE

glossary

BAMBOO SHOOTS the tender shoots of bamboo plants, available in cans; must be drained and rinsed before use.

BARLEY a nutritious grain used in soups and stews. *Hulled barley* is the least processed form of barley and is high in fibre. *Pearl barley* has had the husk discarded and been hulled and polished, much the same as rice.

BAY LEAVES aromatic leaves from the bay tree used to flavour soups, stocks and casseroles.

BEAN SPROUTS also known as bean shoots.

BEANS
black-eyed also known as black-eyed peas.
borlotti also known as roman beans; can be eaten fresh or dried.
green sometimes called french or string beans, this long fresh bean is consumed pod and all.
yellow string also known as wax, french, runner and, incorrectly, butter beans; a yellow-coloured fresh green bean.

BEETROOT also known as red beets or just beets; firm, round root vegetable. Can be eaten raw, grated, in salads; boiled and sliced; or roasted then mashed like potatoes.

BOK CHOY also known as bak choy, pak choi, chinese white cabbage or chinese chard. Has a fresh, mild mustard taste; use both stems and leaves. *Baby bok choy* is smaller and more tender than bok choy.

BROCCOLINI a cross between broccoli and chinese kale. Is milder and sweeter than broccoli. From floret to stem, broccolini is completely edible. Substitute with gai larn or common broccoli.

CAPSICUM also known as bell pepper or, simply, pepper. Can be red, green, yellow, orange or purplish black. Discard seeds and membranes before use.

CARDAMOM one of the world's most expensive spices; has a distinctive aromatic, sweetly rich flavour. Purchase in pod, seed or ground form.

CELERIAC tuberous root with brown skin, white flesh and celery-like flavour.

CHEESE
fetta a crumbly, white goat- or sheep-milk cheese with a sharp salty taste.
goat made from goat milk, has an earthy, strong taste; available in both soft and firm textures, in various shapes and sizes, sometimes rolled in ash or herbs.
ricotta soft white cow milk cheese; roughly translates as "cooked again". Is a sweet, moist cheese with a fat content of around 8.5% and a slightly grainy texture.

CHERVIL also known as cicily; mildly fennel-flavoured herb with curly dark-green leaves.

CHICKPEAS also called garbanzos, hummus or channa; an irregularly round, sandy-coloured legume used extensively in Mediterranean and Latin cooking.

CHINESE CABBAGE also known as peking cabbage, wong bok or petsai. Elongated in shape with pale green, crinkly leaves. Can be shredded or chopped and eaten raw or braised, steamed or stir-fried.

CINNAMON STICK the dried inner bark of the shoots of the cinnamon tree.

COOKING-OIL SPRAY we used a cholesterol-free cooking spray made from canola oil.

CORIANDER also known as cilantro or chinese parsley; bright-green-leafed herb with a pungent flavour. Often stirred into or sprinkled over a dish just before serving for maximum impact. Both the stems and roots are also used in Thai cooking; wash well before chopping.

CURLY ENDIVE also known as frisee, a curly-leafed green vegetable, mainly used in salads.

CURRANTS dried, tiny, almost black raisins so-named after a grape variety that originated in Corinth, Greece.

FENNEL also known as finocchio or anise; eaten raw in salads or braised or fried as a vegetable accompaniment. Also the name given to dried seeds having a licorice flavour.

GAI LARN also known as gai lum, kanah, or chinese kale; appreciated more for its stems than its coarse leaves. Serve steamed and stir-fried, in soups and noodle dishes. Available from Asian food stores and many greengrocers.

GINGER also known as green or root ginger; the thick gnarled root of a tropical plant. Cannot be substituted with ginger powder.

JUICE, FRESH we made our own fresh juice in every recipe.

KAFFIR LIME LEAVES also known as bai magrood; glossy dark green leaves joined end to end to form a rounded hourglass shape. Sold fresh, dried or frozen, the dried leaves are less potent so double the number called for in a recipe if you substitute them for fresh leaves. A strip of fresh lime peel can be substituted for each kaffir lime leaf.

KUMARA Polynesian name of orange-fleshed sweet potato often confused with yam.

KIWI FRUIT also known as chinese gooseberry.

LEBANESE CUCUMBER also known as the european or burpless cucumber; short, slender and thin-skinned.

LEMON GRASS a tall, clumping, lemon-smelling and tasting, sharp-edged grass; the white lower part of each stem is finely chopped and used in Asian cooking or for tea.

LENTILS (red, brown, yellow) dried pulses often identified by and named after their colour.
french green originally from France, these are a small, dark-green, fast-cooking lentils with a delicate flavour.

LYCHEES delicious fruit with a light texture and flavour; peel away rough skin, remove seed and use. Also available in cans.

MANDARIN also known as tangerine; a small, loose-skinned citrus fruit. Segments in a light syrup are available canned.

MANGO tropical fruit with skin colour ranging from green through yellow to deep red. Its fragrant deep yellow flesh surrounds a large flat seed. Mango cheeks in a light syrup are available canned.

MESCLUN mixed baby salad leaves also sold as salad mix or gourmet salad mix; a mixture of assorted young lettuce and other green leaves.

MUSHROOMS
button small, cultivated white mushrooms having a delicate, subtle flavour.
oyster also known as abalone; a grey-white mushroom shaped like a fan. Smooth, with a subtle, oyster-like flavour.
portobello are mature swiss browns. These large, dark brown mushrooms possess a robust, full-bodied flavour, and are ideal for filling or barbecuing.
shiitake when fresh are also known as chinese black, forest or golden oak mushrooms; although cultivated, they have an earthy taste. When dried, are known as donko or dried chinese mushrooms; rehydrate before use.
swiss brown light to dark brown mushrooms with full-bodied flavour. Button or cup mushrooms can be substituted for swiss brown mushrooms.

MUSTARD, AMERICAN a sweet yellow mixture containing mustard seeds, sugar, salt, spices and garlic.

NUTS

almonds flat, pointy-ended nuts with pitted brown shell enclosing a creamy white kernel that is covered by a brown skin.

almonds, flaked paper-thin almond slices.

almonds, slivered small lengthways-cut almond pieces.

pine nuts also known as pignoli; not, in fact, a nut but a small, cream-coloured kernel from pine cones.

pistachio pale green, delicately flavoured nut inside hard, off-white shell. To peel, soak shelled nuts in boiling water for about 5 minutes; drain, pat dry with absorbent paper, then rub skins with cloth to peel.

walnuts a rich, flavourful nut. Store in the refrigerator because of its high oil content.

OIL

grapeseed made from grape seeds. Available from most supermarkets.

olive made from ripened olives. *Extra virgin* and *virgin* are the first and second press, respectively, of the olives, while *extra light* or *light* refers to taste, not fat levels.

peanut pressed from ground peanuts; has high smoke point (capacity to handle high heat without burning).

sesame made from roasted, crushed white sesame seeds.

walnut made from walnuts.

ONIONS

brown and white these are interchangeable. Their pungent flesh adds flavour to a vast range of dishes.

green also known as scallion or, incorrectly, shallot; an immature onion picked before the bulb has formed. Has a bright-green edible stalk.

red also known as red spanish, spanish or bermuda onion; a sweet-flavoured, large, purple-red onion.

shallots also called french shallots, golden shallots or eschalots; small, elongated, brown-skinned members of the onion family. Grows in tight clusters similar to garlic.

spring onions with small white bulbs, long green leaves and narrow green-leafed tops.

PAPAYA also known as pawpaw; a large, pear-shaped red-orange tropical fruit. Sometimes used unripened (green) in cooking.

PARSLEY, FLAT-LEAF known as continental or italian parsley.

PATTY-PAN SQUASH also known as crookneck or custard marrow pumpkins; a round, slightly flat summer squash being yellow to pale-green in colour and having a scalloped edge. Harvested young, it has firm white flesh and distinct flavour.

PEPITAS dried pumpkin seeds.

PEPPERCORNS, BLACK the strongest flavoured of all the peppercorn varieties. They are picked when the berries are not quite ripe, then dried until they shrivel and the skin turns dark brown or black.

POLENTA also known as cornmeal; a flour-like cereal made of dried corn (maize) sold ground in several different textures; also the name of the dish made from it.

PRUNES commercially or sun-dried plums.

RADICCHIO a member of the chicory family. Has dark burgundy leaves and a strong bitter flavour.

RICE, BROWN LONG-GRAIN entire grain with only the inedible outer husk removed; nutritious and high in fibre. Has a nutlike flavour and chewy texture. The elongated grains remain separate when cooked.

ROCKET also known as arugula, rugula and rucola; a peppery-tasting green leaf that can be eaten raw or used in cooking. *Baby rocket leaves* are both smaller and less peppery.

ROLLED OATS oats that have been husked, steamed-softened, flattened and dried.

SESAME SEEDS black and white are the most common, however there are red and brown varieties also. To toast: spread seeds evenly on oven tray, toast in moderate oven briefly.

SILVERBEET also known as seakale or swiss chard. A green-leafed vegetable with sturdy celery-like white stems. Can be used similarly to spinach.

SNOW PEAS also called mange tout. Snow pea tendrils, the growing shoots of the plant, are sold by greengrocers.

SOBA thin spaghetti-like pale brown noodle from Japan made from buckwheat and wheat flour; eaten hot or cold.

SPINACH also known as english spinach and, incorrectly, silverbeet.

SPLIT PEAS also known as field peas. A green or yellow pulse used in soups and stews

SUGAR SNAP PEAS also known as honey snap peas; fresh small pea that can be eaten whole.

SUNFLOWER SEEDS kernels from dried husked sunflower seeds.

SWEDES also known as rutabaga, swedes have a yellow skin and look similar to turnips.

TAHINI sesame seed paste available from Middle-Eastern food stores; most often used in hummus, baba ghanoush and other Lebanese recipes.

TAMARI a thick, dark sauce made mainly from soy beans. Has a distinctive mellow flavour. Is used mainly used as a dipping sauce or for basting. Available from most supermarkets and Asian food stores.

TANGELO a cross between a grapefruit and tangerine; a loose-skinned, juicy, sweetly-tart citrus fruit with few seeds. Is eaten like an orange.

TOFU also known as bean curd, an off-white, custard-like product made from the milk of crushed soy beans; comes fresh (as soft or firm), and processed) as fried or pressed dried sheets). *Silken tofu* refers to the method by which it is made, where it is strained through silk.

TOMATO

cherry also known as tiny tim or tom thumb, small and round.

egg smallish and oval-shaped; also called plum or roma.

TURMERIC also known as kamin; related to galangal and ginger. Must be grated or pounded to release its somewhat acrid aroma and pungent flavour. Fresh turmeric may be substituted with dried turmeric powder (2 teaspoons of ground turmeric plus a teaspoon of sugar for every 20g of fresh turmeric called for in a recipe).

VANILLA EXTRACT vanilla beans infused in alcohol and water.

VINEGAR, CIDER made from fermented apples.

WAKAME a bright-green seaweed, is usually sold in dry form and used in soups, salads and seasonings. Dried wakame must be softened by soaking for about 10 minutes then discarding any hard stems. Wakame can be found in most asian food stores.

WATERCRESS one of the cress family, a large group of peppery greens used raw in salads, dips and sandwiches, or cooked in soups. Highly perishable, so must be used as soon as possible after purchase.

YOGURT we used either sheep- or goat-milk yogurt in this book.

ZUCCHINI also called courgette. A member of the squash family, having edible flowers.

index

GENERAL INDEX

breathing 14
cleaning up 6
detox(ing)
  after 18
  coming out of 18
  do you need to detox? 5
  eating out during 17
  exercise and 10
  foods to avoid during 8
  hero foods 6
  how you know you need to 5
  other foods 8
  pampering during 13
  pamper yourself 11
  possible side effects of 15
  preparing to 6
  when to – and when not to 5
  why you need to 4
  your emotions 16
eating out during detox 17
emotions, detoxing your 16
exercise and detox 10
foods
  excellent detox 8
  hero detox 6
  menu plans 20
  to avoid 8
getting the balance right 10
H20 10
herbal teas 16
menu plans 20
  one-day mono-food detox 20
  one weekend detox 20
  seven-day detox 21
  two-week detox 22
pamper yourself 11
  aromatherapy 11
  bath blends 13
  body pampering
    during detox 13
  dry body brushing and
    an Epsom Salts bath 11
  essential oils 11
  facials 14
  massage 14
  other hydrotherapy
    treatments 13
  reflexology 13
preparing to detox 6
reducing toxic overload,
  more ways to 18
side effects of
  detoxing, possible 15
teas, herbal 16
toxic overload, more ways
  to reduce 18

RECIPE INDEX

dips
  beetroot dip 76
  carrot dip 76
  hummus 77
  raita 77
fish
  steamed asian bream 34
  grilled blue-eye with
    gai larn 36
  poached flathead with
    herb salad 35
fruit dishes
  apple and blueberry muesli 32
  apple and pear compote
    with dates 104
  banana with passionfruit 109
  banana with passionfruit
    yogurt 107
  blood plums with honey
    and cardamon yogurt 110
  cherries and yogurt 111
  figs with sheep-milk
    yogurt and honey 108
  four-fruit combo 106
  kiwi fruit, lychee and
    lime salad 108
  lychees with passionfruit 109
  macerated fruits 106
  mango cheeks with
    lime wedges 111
  papaya with passionfruit
    and lime 107
  porridge with poached
    pears and blueberries 26
  stewed prunes with orange 110
juices
  apple and celery 45
  apple and pear 44
  beetroot, carrot and
    spinach 43
  carrot, ginger
    and silverbeet 49
  ginger, orange
    and pineapple 46
  grapefruit and
    blood orange 47
  kiwi fruit and green grape 47
  mandarin 46
  mango and grapefruit 45
  mixed berry 42
  orange and ginger 42
  orange, carrot and celery 48
  orange, carrot and ginger 49
  orange, mango
    and strawberry 48
  peach, apple and strawberry 40
  pear and ginger 48
  pear and grape 45
  pineapple, ginger and mint 46

  pineapple, orange
    and strawberry 43
  raspberry and peach 42
  silverbeet, apple and celery 44
  strawberry and papaya 40
  tangelo and ginger 47
  watercress, beetroot
    and celery 40
  watermelon and mint 43
milk drinks
  almond milk 114
  banana soy smoothie 49
  strawberry, honey
    and soy smoothie 44
salads
  asparagus caesar 24
  baked beetroot with cannellini
    beans, fetta and mint 103
  borlotti beans, brown rice
    and almond 93
  chickpea patties with tomato
    and cucumber salad 73
  chickpea, watercress
    and capsicum 90
  cos, snow pea and
    roasted celeriac 89
  greek 84
  green vegetable, with american
    mustard dressing 78
  kiwi, lychee and lime salad 108
  lamb's lettuce with
    pecans and orange 81
  grilled asparagus with
    warm tomato dressing 97
  mixed bean 31
  orange, fennel and almond 82
  pan-fried tofu with
    vietnamese coleslaw 86
  pear, spinach, walnut
    and celery 95
  pearl barley 88
  poached flathead with herb 35
  potato and bean with
    lemon yogurt dressing 85
  potato and asparagus with
    yogurt and mint dressing 91
  roasted egg tomatoes
    with barley 94
  roasted pumpkin,
    pecan and fetta 101
  soba with seaweed,
    ginger and vegetables 98
  spinach and zucchini
    with yogurt hummus 83
  thai soy bean with grapes
    and pink grapefruit 96
  tomato and avocado
    with tofu pesto 100
  white bean 27

sandwiches/wrap
  open rye sandwich 30
  lavash wrap 29
  salad, goat cheese and
    pecan sandwich 28
broth/soups/stock
  asian broth 52
  leek and potato soup 55
  lentil and vegetable soup 59
  pumpkin and kumara soup 56
  roasted tomato and
    capsicum soup 53
  vegetable and soba soup 57
  vegetable soup 54
  vegetable stock 50
teas and hot drinks
  cardamom and
    chamomile tea 114
  cinnamon and orange tea 115
  grapefruit water, hot 112
  ginger tea 115
  lemon grass and
    kaffir lime leaf tea 114
  lemon water, hot 112
  mint tea 115
vegetable dishes
  baked potato with
    guacamole 68
  black-eyed beans with kumara,
    shallots and garlic 64
  brown rice pilaf 75
  brown rice with vegetables
    and tahini dressing 67
  chickpea patties with tomato
    and cucumber salad 73
  dahl with vegetables 66
  eggplant with salsa fresca 71
  grilled asparagus with
    warm tomato dressing 97
  leek, goat cheese and
    brown lentil bake 69
  oven-roasted ratatouille
    with almond gremolata 39
  ratatouille 63
  roasted cherry tomatoes,
    broccolini and pepitas 62
  roasted root vegetables
    with yogurt 70
  roasted vegetable stack 65
  stir-fried asian greens
    with mixed mushrooms 72
  stir-fried asian greens
    with tofu 60
  stir-fried tofu with vegetables
    and lemon grass 74
  vegetable and white
    bean stew 37
  vegetable stir-fry 33

facts + figures

Wherever you live, you'll be able to use our recipes with the help of these easy-to-follow conversions. While these conversions are approximate only, the difference between an exact and the approximate conversion of various liquid and dry measures is minimal and will not affect your cooking results.

LIQUID MEASURES

METRIC	IMPERIAL
30ml	1 fluid oz
60ml	2 fluid oz
100ml	3 fluid oz
125ml	4 fluid oz
150ml	5 fluid oz (¼ pint/1 gill)
190ml	6 fluid oz
250ml	8 fluid oz
300ml	10 fluid oz (½ pint)
500ml	16 fluid oz
600ml	20 fluid oz (1 pint)
1000ml (1 litre)	1¾ pints

MEASURING EQUIPMENT

The difference between one country's measuring cups and another's is, at most, within a 2 or 3 teaspoon variance. (For the record, one Australian metric measuring cup holds approximately 250ml.) The most accurate way of measuring dry ingredients is to weigh them. When measuring liquids, use a clear glass or plastic jug with the metric markings. (One Australian metric tablespoon holds 20ml; one Australian metric teaspoon holds 5ml.)

DRY MEASURES

METRIC	IMPERIAL
15g	½oz
30g	1oz
60g	2oz
90g	3oz
125g	4oz (¼lb)
155g	5oz
185g	6oz
220g	7oz
250g	8oz (½lb)
280g	9oz
315g	10oz
345g	11oz
375g	12oz (¾lb)
410g	13oz
440g	14oz
470g	15oz
500g	16oz (1lb)
750g	24oz (1½lb)
1kg	32oz (2lb)

HELPFUL MEASURES

METRIC	IMPERIAL
3mm	⅛in
6mm	¼in
1cm	½in
2cm	¾in
2.5cm	1in
5cm	2in
6cm	2½in
8cm	3in
10cm	4in
13cm	5in
15cm	6in
18cm	7in
20cm	8in
23cm	9in
25cm	10in
28cm	11in
30cm	12in (1ft)

HOW TO MEASURE

When using graduated metric measuring cups, shake dry ingredients loosely into the appropriate cup. Do not tap the cup on a bench or tightly pack the ingredients unless directed to do so. Level top of measuring cups and measuring spoons with a knife. When measuring liquids, place a clear glass or plastic jug with metric markings on a flat surface to check accuracy at eye level.

Note: North America, NZ and the UK use 15ml tablespoons. All cup and spoon measurements are level.

We use large eggs having an average weight of 60g.

OVEN TEMPERATURES

These oven temperatures are only a guide for conventional ovens.
For fan-forced ovens, check the manufacturer's manual.

	°C (CELSIUS)	°F (FAHRENHEIT)	GAS MARK
Very slow	120	250	½
Slow	150	275-300	1-2
Moderately slow	160	325	3
Moderate	180	350-375	4-5
Moderately hot	200	400	6
Hot	220	425-450	7-8
Very hot	240	475	9

Looking after **your interest...**

Keep your ACP cookbooks clean, tidy and within easy reach with a book holder designed to hold up to 12 books. Plus you can follow our recipes perfectly with a set of accurate measuring cups and spoons, as used by *The Australian Women's Weekly* Test Kitchen.

To order

Mail or fax Photocopy and complete the coupon below and post to ACP Books Reader Offer, ACP Publishing, GPO Box 4967, Sydney NSW 2001, or fax to (02) 9267 4967.

Phone Have your credit card details ready, then phone 136 116 (Mon-Fri, 8.00am-6.00pm; Sat, 8.00am-6.00pm).

Price

Book Holder

Australia: $13.10 (incl. GST).
Elsewhere: $A21.95.

Metric Measuring Set

Australia: $6.50 (incl. GST).
New Zealand: $A8.00.
Elsewhere: $A9.95.

Prices include postage and handling. This offer is available in all countries.

Payment

Australian residents

We accept the credit cards listed on the coupon, money orders and cheques.

Overseas residents

We accept the credit cards listed on the coupon, drafts in $A drawn on an Australian bank, and also UK, NZ and US cheques in the currency of the country of issue. Credit card charges are at the exchange rate current at the time of payment.

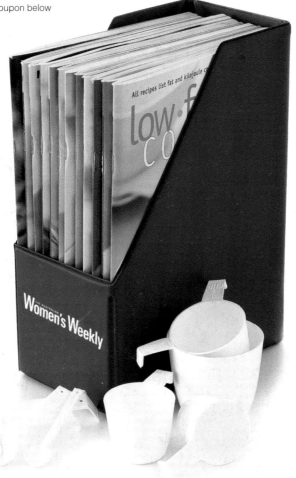

Photocopy and complete coupon below

☐ **Book Holder**

☐ **Metric Measuring Set**
  Please indicate number(s) required.

Mr/Mrs/Ms _____

Address _____

_____

Postcode _____ Country _____

Ph: Business hours ( ) _____

I enclose my cheque/money order for $ _____ payable to ACP Publishing.

OR: please charge my

☐ Bankcard ☐ Visa ☐ Mastercard

☐ Diners Club ☐ American Express

Card number

Expiry date ____ /____

Cardholder's signature _____

Please allow up to 30 days delivery within Australia. Allow up to 6 weeks for overseas deliveries. Both offers expire 31/12/06. HLD06

Test Kitchen
Food director *Pamela Clark*
Food editor *Karen Hammial*
Assistant food editor *Amira Georgy*
Test Kitchen manager *Cathie Lonnie*
Home economists *Arianne Bradshaw, Nicole Jennings, Elizabeth Macri, Sharon Reeve, Susie Riggall, Kirrily Smith, Rebecca Squadrito, Kellie Thomas, Helen Webster*
Nutritional information *Angela Muscat*

ACP Books
Editorial director *Susan Tomnay*
Creative director *Hieu Chi Nguyen*
Senior editor *Wendy Bryant*
Designer *Corey Butler*
Contributing writer *Helen Hawkes*
Sales director *Brian Cearnes*
Marketing director *Matt Dominello*
Brand manager *Renée Crea*
Production manager *Carol Currie*
Chief executive officer *John Alexander*
Group publisher *Pat Ingram*
Publisher *Sue Wannan*
Editorial director (AWW) *Deborah Thomas*

Produced by ACP Books, Sydney.
Printed by Times Printers, Singapore.
Published by ACP Publishing Pty Limited, 54 Park St, Sydney; GPO Box 4088, Sydney, NSW 2001.
Ph: (02) 9282 8618 Fax: (02) 9267 9438.
acpbooks@acp.com.au
www.acpbooks.com.au
To order books, phone 136 116.
Send recipe enquiries to:
recipeenquiries@acp.com.au
RIGHTS ENQUIRIES
Laura Bamford, Director ACP Books.
lbamford@acplon.co.uk
Ph: +44 (207) 812 6526
AUSTRALIA: Distributed by Network Services, GPO Box 4088, Sydney, NSW 2001.
Ph: (02) 9282 8777 Fax: (02) 9264 3278.
UNITED KINGDOM: Distributed by Australian Consolidated Press (UK), Moulton Park Business Centre, Red House Rd, Moulton Park, Northampton, NN3 6AQ.
Ph: (01604) 497531 Fax: (01604) 497533
acpukltd@aol.com
CANADA: Distributed by Whitecap Books Ltd, 351 Lynn Ave, North Vancouver, BC, V7J 2C4.
Ph: (604) 980 9852 Fax: (604) 980 8197
customerservice@whitecap.ca
www.whitecap.ca
NEW ZEALAND: Distributed by Netlink Distribution Company, ACP Media Centre, Cnr Fanshawe and Beaumont Streets, Westhaven, Auckland.
PO Box 47906, Ponsonby, Auckland, NZ.
Ph: (09) 366 9966 Fax: 0800 277 412
ask@ndcnz.co.nz
SOUTH AFRICA: Distributed by PSD Promotions, 30 Diesel Road Isando, Gauteng Johannesburg.
PO Box 1175, Isando 1600, Gauteng Johannesburg.
Ph: (2711) 392 6065/6/7
Fax: (2711) 392 6079/80
orders@psdprom.co.za

Clark, Pamela.
The Australian Women's Weekly detox.
Includes index.
ISBN 1 86396 470 3.
1. Cookery. 2. Detoxification (Health)
I. Title. II Title: Australian Women's Weekly.

641.563
© ACP Publishing Pty Limited 2005
ABN 18 053 273 546